HEALING HANDS
HEALING WORDS

HEALING HANDS
HEALING WORDS
You can help healing happen

by

Ray Cullis

ThreeCatsPub

Disclaimer

The information in this book is not intended to replace medical treatment or advice. You should consult your physician regarding any general or specific physical symptoms. The author and publisher disclaim any responsibility for adverse effects resulting from information in this book.

First Edition Copyright ©1998 by Raymond W. Cullis

2nd Edition Copyright ©2020 by Raymond W. Cullis

Δ

This book was originally published in 1998 by
A.R.E. Press, 215 67th Street, Virginia Beach, Va. 23451-2061

CONTENTS

Acknowledgments

(1998)

Thanks to Susan Phillips and staff at the Yaupon Beach branch of the Brunswick County (NC) Public Library for use of their computers, for tutoring in WordPerfect, and for their cheerful patience.

Several people in Nevada, Missouri, were most willing to provide, or direct me to information about Sidney A. Weltmer and the Weltmer Institute. My gratitude to them.

My appreciation also to Jean Marcley, a professional counselor and hypnotherapist who gave me advice for one of the relaxation methods described in Chapter 5.

(2019)

I wish to thank the Brunswick Arts Council of Brunswick County, NC for grant money to purchase the computer and software I used in the production of the current edition of this book, and other books that I have written.

Thanks also to my friend Jacqueline DeGroot for the final proofreading of this new edition of *Healing Hands Healing Words*.

PREFACE

—

Q. Anyone you would suggest to give these (healing treatments)?

A. Of course, better one who is versed in such; but anyone that will take the time would be very well.

Edgar Cayce reading 543-26

You can help healing happen. It is the purpose of this book to explain why this is possible and to provide you with a specific healing technique from the Edgar Cayce psychic readings and from Sidney A. Weltmer.

The Cayce readings interpret how healing occurs within the body from a spiritual perspective. They also tell us how we can help such healing happen. Actually, only God heals. We can, however, facilitate healing by creating an environment conducive to healing. In creating such conditions we actually participate in the healing process.

> *To each individual soul has been given the privilege, yea the opportunity, to become a co-worker with the Lord among his brethern.* (3019-1)

This book is written for the layperson, anyone who seeks to supplement—not substitute—orthodox medical care with a spiritual, non-invasive approach to healing physical ailments of friends and loved ones.

For interested health professionals I have included an addendum they may find useful in their practice.

The first section of this book addresses the nature of healing as it applies to the spiritual approach and its influence in healing. Here is information from the Cayce readings on the body's divine nature, its self-healing birthright, and the role of the subconscious in healing. These first three chapters lay groundwork intended to strengthen one's faith in the healing technique taught in the second part of the book. Christ said, *"...thy faith has made thee whole."* (Matt. 9:22) In gaining understanding of this spiritual healing process we can come to believe in it.

Part II of this book details the specific healing technique which Cayce referred to in reading 300-1 as *"suggestive magnetic treatments or therapeutics."* Many times he recommended this simple healing method which combines what he called the "electromagnetic" energy of the hands with the power of suggestion to motivate the spontaneous healing of which all bodies are inherently capable. The power of suggestion referred to here is not hypnotism. Rather, it is the repeating of simple verbal statements or affirmations to a person while he or she is in a relaxed, receptive state. This relaxed state makes it possible for the patient, who may be fearful and doubtful of the outcome of his condition, to accept and believe the healing suggestion.

The role of both the electromagnetic energy of the hands and verbal suggestions are to raise the vibrations necessary for healing to begin within the patient or subject. It is somewhat similar to jump-starting a car or priming a pump.

I have found that while these methods are simple, the preparation necessary to create the healing attitude can be mentally and physically demanding, yet rewarding. For, with sincere effort the spiritual benefits to the healer are great.

> ...for in being such a channel there comes to such individuals those of blessings that few may ever know. (Cayce reading 295-6)

It is the spirit of unselfish desire to help others, and the willingness to credit God with any healing, that raises our own spiritual state and consciousness.

My personal interest in healing began in the early 1970s. At that time I was massage therapist at A.R.E. Therapy Department in Virginia Beach and often researched the Edgar Cayce readings on massage. It was then that I discovered Cayce's references to Sidney Weltmer and magnetic healing and suggestion.

In the past few years I've become more interested in this form of spiritual healing. This book is the result of my own desire to learn more about suggestive magnetic therapy and to make the information available to others.

~Ray Cullis, 1997

Part I

FOUNDATIONS FOR HEALING

1

WHO CAN HEAL?

———

...there should be some individual chosen, in whom the body has confidence, that would use a thirty minute to an hour period each day for reading, meditating, praying with the body; and using at the same time the magnetic healing treatment... (Edgar Cayce reading 3035-1)

The good doctor bent over her patient, assessing the damage caused by the accident. Then, adjusting the gadget in her hand, she held it an inch or so above the wound for a few seconds and watched the injury heal before her eyes. Commonplace procedure on *Star Trek: the Next Generation,* but one that's far off in the future! What exactly did the gadget do—that wonder of futuristic technology? It changed the vibrations of the atoms within the injured body to access the creative energies of the universe, allowing the body to heal itself.

This is not as extraordinary as we might think. Consider this: The Edgar Cayce readings tell us that healing is spontaneous, occurring from within, and that it happens by attuning the body's vibrations to those of the Creator—God.

Cayce once was asked if healing is a gift or a talent developed in past lives. "Both," he replied. *"All force, all power, comes from the same source."* (262-3)

Some who received readings from Cayce were told that they had healing experience from the time Christ:

The entity was among those of the household of the jailer whom Paul aided when he was released from prison... the entity then, as the wife of the jailer, made profession of the faith and became active as a healer.

Hence the entity will find in itself today, if there is the renewing of the spiritual influences from within, the laying on of hands or the magnetic treatment will be very effective under the hands of this entity. (3478-2)

The ability to heal could have originated even further back in time, even to unrecorded history. In a reading for one woman she was told her healing ability dated back to Atlantis, *"... for the entity then was a daughter of one in authority in Atlantis, and thus a priestess...there was the ability to aid by the very high vibrations of the body itself... And the entity has healing in its hands in the present."* (2655-1)

We should be so fortunate as to already have the ability to heal. And we do. We all do! Undeveloped as it may be, it is nonetheless inborn in us all. We may not have the talent from past lives, but we are born with mind and body – all the equipment we need to be healers. We have but to learn to use them for healing just as we have to learn anything for which we have potential. Even those among us with past life healing experience may need to reawaken their ability by spiritual self-renewal. Something we all need to do frequently if not daily, anyway. Think of that, it is doubly rewarding; we grow by our renewed and continued spiritual involvement, while at the same time being a channel of hope and help to others. If our purposes and motives are unselfish, we cannot learn to heal without growing spiritually.

(Q) How can I best develop the magnetic power for healing?

(A) First understanding self; and do not become mechanical or rote in action. Rather be the growth as the spirit moves self, as the understanding comes – but much may be accomplished through these channels. (281-9)

As we seek to grow spiritually, attempting to become channels for healing, we are entering sacred ground. For we come in contact with the First Cause, God, as we raise our consciousness and seek to raise the vibrations in another to facilitate healing. This is what re-creation, regeneration—what healing is all about. The attuning of self to the awesome fact that God is—that God's very nature is creative and constructive in all his activities – is to be in touch with the Creator and sustaining force of life. When we touch the hem of his garment, when we raise our consciousness to God's realm, so do we make ourselves channels of his energies, his vibrations, which are healing by their very nature.

Edgar Cayce tells us that all methods of healing are spiritual in that, when successful, they reach or move the divine within us to bring about healing. He put it this way, *"... from whence comes the healing? Whether there is administered a drug, a correcting or an ad-justment of a subluxation, or the alleviating of a strain upon the muscles, or the revivifying through electrical forces; they are <u>one</u>, and the healing comes from <u>within</u>."*(969-1) Regardless of whether it is orthodox medicine, an alternative healing approach, or a religious/spiritual approach, for healing to happen each must activate that part of us which is self-healing. It is the spiritual nature within us which must be stirred or moved.

That not all can be healed by the same method is a long-known fact. It depends on the consciousness of each individual as to what method will work for him or her. *"Not by the method does the healing come, though the consciousness of the individual is such that this or that method <u>is</u> the one that is more effective in the individual case in arousing the forces from within,"* Cayce continued in reading 969-1.

By faith we are healed, Christ said. And so, even he used different methods to heal. For some he used only the spoken word, others he touched with his hands, and he used still other methods to heal depending on the individual seeking help. But he most often used both the power of his words and the transforming energy of his hands to heal. And even Christ admitted that it was not he who did the work, rather, it was God within him. So may we become co-workers with him; *"He that believeth on me, the works that I do shall he do also...because I go unto my Father."* (John 14:12)

It is inspiring to learn that we can facilitate healing ourselves, not with some man-made instrument, but with the body and the mind which our Creator has given us. With our minds we can encourage healing to happen by the use of suggestion and positive affirmations. With our bodies we can direst healing energy through our hands to others. Using both of these simultaneously is the healing method Edgar Cayce called "suggestive magnetic treatments or therapeutics." Cayce recommended this technique many times, sometimes using slightly different words for the same treatment:

(Q) What should be done for the trouble in my head?
(A) This is mostly reflex. The adjustments made
Osteopathically...will relieve these tensions that are left after the corrections are made through the magnetic and suggestive treatments. (3691-1)

Again, Cayce emphasized that both forms of healing be used together:

(Q) Should all the same treatments be continued?
(A) All the same treatments, and these for the magnetic and suggestive force combined. (1371-2)

Other times he described the treatment in a way less obvious to the casual researcher:

Then, in the present, there may be either the increase of the circulation by magnetic influences or through the application of heat, with the vibrations of electrical forces in the violet ray over the area, or through the combined application of these with suggestion. (294-165)

The fact that the Cayce readings did not refer to the technique by one particular name in all the readings that recommended the treatment may have contributed to the obscurity of the therapy. Actually, suggestive magnetic therapy was widely accepted and practiced in the first third of this century, thanks to a man named Sidney A.

Weltmer. It was the school and treatment center founded by Weltmer that Cayce referred to in reading number 5702 -1: *"Such may be found in that treatment as may be accorded by A. C. Lane...or by the Weltmer Institute at Nevada, Missouri."*

Sidney Wilmer devoted the last half of his life to the practice and teaching of suggestive magnetic therapy though he did not use exactly that name for his healing method. He referred to it as "suggestive therapeutics" at times and other times simply as magnetic healing. Still, his method employs a combination of both.

Weltmer was born in the 1850s. In his early years he was a student of mesmerism, studied various spiritual philosophies including those of the Orient, and for a time considered becoming a medical doctor. As a teenager, because of the demand for schoolteachers, he quickly moved from being a student to becoming a teacher himself. His speaking ability and his spiritual interests led him to become a licensed minister at age nineteen.

After a few years he quit the ministry, saying he would not preach again until he learned to heal, as he believed Jesus meant people to do. His study of the Scriptures and healing methods of his day culminated in his discovery of suggestion as a powerful healing tool. The use of the hands for healing, he determined, was also a form of suggestion, though he understood that healing energies or vibrations flowed through the hands.

After several years of continued study and practice, his methods became very well established in his mind and formed his healing philosophy. Based on his successful healing experience, he founded the Weltmer Institute in 1897.

The Institute, re-chartered in 1906 as the Weltmer Institute of Suggestive Therapeutics Company, was a four-year school. Its curriculum included many of the same courses offered in medical schools at that time. In addition, the four-year course included such subjects as "Experimental Psychology and Psychic Research," "Suggestive Therapeutics," hypnotism, and a course in massage.

While the Institute functioned as a school, it was also a highly successful treatment facility. By 1910 the school's records showed treatment of over one hundred fifty thousand people annually. Most of these people came for treatment after being abandoned as incurable by others, according to Weltmer.

Sidney Weltmer believed that healing could be learned, and that anyone could heal as he did if one knew what he did. He proved that through his students at the Institution; they became well educated, licensed practitioners of suggestive therapeutics. He also taught many others his philosophy and healing method through a mail correspondence course.

It was Weltmer's way to teach thoroughly what he felt his students should know to become proficient healers.

He taught his students to heal with specific techniques for various ailments. While this is fine for healthcare professionals, we will use more general methods for all ailments. Edgar Cayce's prerequisites for healing with suggestive magnetic therapeutics are much more lenient. (Part II will have more on the practical application of this healing technique.)

How are we to know if we would be effective healers, or facilitators for healing? Cayce is a big help in answering this question. Many who received readings from him asked whom they should use for magnetic healing. Surprisingly, Cayce usually recommended people with no particular talent for healing. Indeed, he seldom mentioned someone by name to do suggestive magnetic healing. Instead, those he recommended were to have no special qualifications other than an attitude conducive to healing and adequate physical energy.

...The magnetic forces that we have indicated heretofore, if these are applied in a consistent manner with the activities in the mental [suggestion], in eradicating fear, doubt, from the thinking of the body – and we will continue improvements.

(Q) Who should give the magnetic treatment?

(A) Anyone that will do the same consistently and conscientiously.

(Q) Would the husband [853] be a suitable person?

(A) He would be a very suitable person. This should be given...with that feeling, that attitude of giving strength of self to make for the activities through the affected portions. (264-44)

Having the right attitude for healing sometimes just comes naturally because of family ties. Also the healing vibrations may be more forthcoming from one who has previously been helped by the subject, as in case 2187-1: *"Have one of those who has been aided or helped by the activities of this body (younger would be better, to be sure, but sufficiently old to know the intent and purpose of such), to sit by the body and give the constant hand magnetic treatment...Of course, the one who makes the application may be changed from time to time – just so it is one who has been aided by the body and is not too old of a person, but one sufficiently minded to know the intent and purpose of such."*

At times Casey did recommend a particular person. In the following case it was someone whom he had earlier given a reading for:

(Q) Would you recommend anyone for the healing work with the hands...?

(A) One who is very close to the body. Such as [1662] would be very good...

He has the necessary ability. Also he has the ability to direct such applications by suggestion to the body so as to become a helpful influence. (2474-1)

Cayce was not without a sense of humor in answering questions put to him while he was in the trance state. He seemed to know there were plenty of people who could do suggestive magnetic treatments and, in this case, left it up to the questioner to find one:

(Q) Mr. Cayce, how will you determine who has this magnetic force?
(A) There are thousands of them. Just find one.
(Q) Mr. Cayce, this body does not know of any such person who could do this work.
(A) No fault of ours here. (5708-1)

We learn from the readings that it takes a certain amount of energy, a focused, loving attitude, and – for giving the suggestions—an ability to verbalize the healing affirmation. As we will note in Chapter 7, the suggestions that are given in suggestive magnetic therapy are short and repeated only a few times during a treatment, rather than continuously. One need not be a tireless talker as Cayce stressed in reading 5636-1: *"The magnetic treatments are a low form of body electrical vibration. Hence should be given by a body with a good deal of energy, vitality, but not one that would talk the person to death while giving it to him!"*

The technique of suggestive magnetic therapy, simply put, involves getting the subject into a relaxed state, then using the power of suggestion and energy through the hands to establish an environment in which healing can happen. Sidney Weltmer's approach involved three main elements: intention, suggestion, and the laying on of hands. Intention is the purpose, the healing thoughts focused upon by the healer; suggestion, the verbalized affirmation employed to reach the sub-conscious mind; laying on of hands, the method used to send electro-magnetic energy which help raise the subject's own vibrations.

One of Casey's readings, number 3619-1, recommended treatment practically identical to the Weltmer method: *"As we find here, the relaxing of the body by or through suggestions made as to almost hypnotize the body will help. This should be done by the power of suggestion at the same time that applications would be made for magnetic healing. This may be done by the very close associates of the body..."*

It is important to understand that suggestive magnetic therapy does *not* involve hypnosis. Cayce did recommend hypnosis many times. He often referred to it simply as suggestion. However, he also used the word "suggestion" in much more general terms, even to suggestion as is used in everyday conversation. Therefore, the Edgar Cayce readings must be closely scrutinized to determine when he used the word to mean hypnosis or the passive relaxed state sought for this healing method.

Weltmer's technique was to put the subject into a very relaxed, passive attitude, not hypnosis. He claimed from his long experience in healing that, while the hypnotic state often affected the patient's condition more rapidly, the *"...cures effected through suggestion in the passive condition are far more permanent than the cures effected through the hypnotic condition."* His claim came from over thirty years of practicing suggestive therapeutics, as he called it.

The role of the subconscious in healing is discussed in Chapter 3. Suggestion is more fully covered there as well as in Chapter Seven.

As we began using this healing method, we will soon find that our purpose must be unselfish and our efforts not merely on the mental and spiritual levels. The raising of our own vibrations requires that we attune ourselves also on the physical level, this often being a major challenge for many of us. Cayce tells us, *"... there are the needs for the purging of the body, of mind; so that through the mind – and the laying on of hands – the entity may bring to others that of health, hope and understanding."* (2329-3)

Attunement is most likely achieved when we are able to treat our bodies as the temple of the living God in which He has promised to meet us; that is, if we can purify our bodies to the best of our abilities by eating healthy foods, exercising, and getting adequate sleep, we are much more likely to be able to attune ourselves mentally and spiritually to our Creator.

It is well to keep in mind that how we treat our physical bodies does affect our healing potential. It is our responsibility to keep it in the best condition possible. Again, Cayce tells us all three aspects of self must be prepared for that healing experience:

The entity finds itself a body, a mind, a soul. The entity has urges that are physical, mental, spiritual. If the entity has attuned self to the infinite – in spirit or in soul, and in mind and body – so that the source of supply allows energies to come through the body, these may be applied through the activities of the body by suggestion as well as through radiation from the magnetism of the body itself. (3068-1)

So who can heal? *You* can. It requires only interest, preparation, practice, and spiritual orientation. Naturally, for some it will be easy, and they may have good results from their efforts in the very beginning. Those of us who find it more difficult and challenging to prepare ourselves spiritually, mentally, and physically may, in the long run, find the greatest personal growth. While the purpose of becoming facilitators for healing is to help others, we simply cannot do so without growing spiritually in the process. Those who find it most difficult may also have the most growth. It is a continual process, not a goal to be reached. Once we overcome one stepping stone, we are thus prepared for even greater ones. Such is the nature of spiritual progress.

Therefore, do not be discouraged if at first it is difficult. If you have much to overcome, you will also have greater wisdom and peace when you have done so. The practice of suggestive magnetic therapy is simple. It is the spiritual, mental, and physical preparation that is the challenge. That challenge is easiest met when we look to God as our guide, strength, constant companion, and as the healer we seek to serve.

In preparation for healing, the following Cayce reading is both inspiring and instructional – so much so that the entire reading is quoted here. You may find it worth referring to often for guidance as you continue your practice and study of healing:

In giving advice or counsel respecting spiritual healing, who is to judge as to whether correct methods are used or not? This comes much as the question that was asked of the Master when the brother asked, "make my brother divide the inheritance with me." His answer: "who made me a judge among men?"

There is one judge – that is the Divine within self. And the judgment itself is "My spirit beareth witness with His spirit."

To each individual soul has been given the privilege, yea the opportunity, to become a co-worker with the Lord among his brethren. And it must depend upon the individual entity as to what power, what influence, is accredited with the individual's power of concentration and of aid to others.

As recorded when individuals saw Paul heal those individuals at Laodicea, even by the sending of a kerchief or by the laying on of hands – and there was the attempt of others to apply the same character, or to produce the same manifestation – there was the speaking out of those forces that would be hindered, in saying: "Jesus we know. Paul we know. But who art thou?"

There is within each individual entity the soul, the mind, the body. By those rituals within self, and the magnetic power, there may be produced that which may have an influence upon others. For, as the master gave, "he that received a profit in the name of a prophet receives a prophet's reward."

That does not indicate as to whether such is done to the glory of self, to the honor of the individual, or to the glory and honor of God. For, it is the ability of each soul, by faith, to receive that as may be a pronouncement from another soul. This is part of the universal law.

Yet the promise has been, "I go to the Father – and greater things ye shall do in my name. For I will bear witness of you – that love me and keep my commandments."

This is the sure way, the pure way – this is the way individuals may so attune their bodies, their minds, their souls, to be healers, to be interpreters, to be ministers, to be various channels of his blessing to others.

These choose thou. As to whether the spirits bear witness with thee – these are to be judged by thine own interpretation of the results obtained. For as he hath given, 'by their fruits you shall know them.'

"Many come and in the last day declare, 'Did we not in thy name cast out demons? Did we not heal the sick?' And I will declare, depart from me – I never knew you."

Hence the answer to each soul, as it applies self in a service to others, must be within self. For, as the lawgiver declared, "Today there is set before thee good and evil. Choose thou." And, "today there is life and death, and he that would save his life shall lose it; but he that shall lose his life in my name, for my name, the same shall find it. For I came," saith He, "that ye might have life and have it more abundantly."

For He is life, the truth, the way. In Him ye may accomplish much. In thyself you may accomplish, but to who's undoing?

Let that mind be in thee, then, that was in the Christ, Jesus, who thought it not robbery to make Himself equal with God, but made Himself of no estate; that ye through Him might know the way – to the Father.

Analyze, then, thyself; thy purposes, thy hopes, thy joys. If thy life manifests the fruit of the spirit—love, patience, joy, long-suffering, brotherly love, kindness—then ye are in that way. If it manifests avarice, hate, jealousy, backbiting, ye know the end. For there is no other name given under heaven whereby men may be saved.

Who then, healeth all thy illnesses? Who wipeth away the tears? Who maketh the heart glad? Who bringth peace and contentment in the soul?"

He that is the Prince of Peace; He that is the light, the way, the truth. In Him there is no faltering; no fault, no condemnation found in others.

Keep the faith. We are through. (3019-1)

We are all on a spiritual pilgrimage back to God. By learning to facilitate healing—by becoming co-workers with God—that journey is enhanced. Those that we help along the way are not indebted to us, they are our benefactors. For we grow to heaven leaning on the arm and the shoulder of those we have helped in consciousness, to paraphrase Edgar Cayce.

May prayer, meditation, intuition, and common sense guide you on your journey.

2

HOW HEALING HAPPENS

———

Practically all of us have experienced physical healing. A scratch, a scrape, a minor cut hardly concerns us. For we know that within a few days the wound will heal with little or no help from us. This is the miracle of spontaneous healing—the body healing itself from within.

We take this self-healing capacity of our bodies for granted. All living things have this ability to heal. All living things are permeated with the life force which we call God. And God is ever creating, regenerating, and mending living things.

The difference between living and inanimate things is obvious. An automobile, if it is dented or has its engine malfunction, will remain that way until repaired. It cannot repair itself. And unless it is repaired, rust will eventually set in and take its toll on the car. Without help from humans the car would never "get better." Its condition would continue to deteriorate until it became irreparable and useless.

We humans are blessed. If we break an arm, a doctor can set the bone in its proper position and protect it with a splint or cast while it heals. The doctor does not heal the bone. It heals itself. All the doctor can do is to make conditions favorable for healing to happen. If conditions are right, the life force will perform its natural function and mend the broken bone.

Healing for a particular ailment may come in a number of different ways. Traditional medicine, alternative medicine, or spiritual healing may affect a cure either alone or in addition to one or both of the other approaches.

A person with a particular ailment may be healed by using one method while another person with the same problem may find healing from a different method.

Whatever the treatment, if it is to facilitate healing it must, according to Cayce, cause a reaction in the body at a very deep level; that is, in the atoms of the body. It is at this level that creation happens. It is also in the atoms that disharmony first appears. When enough atoms are out of sync with the creative energy, that is, if their vibrations are other than creative, they can have a destructive effect on the body at the molecular level. If the destructive vibrations continue to multiply from atoms and molecules to cells, then noticeable effects begin to be registered by the body. This can happen very rapidly—immediately in the case of an accident or injury—or it may occur slowly over a long period of time.

Attitudes and Healing

No matter what the cause of a physical problem and regardless how serious it may be, one of the most constructive things and ailing person can do is to believe that he or she can be healed. Sidney Weltmer noted that of the patients who came to him over the years, those who were most likely to be healed were easy to identify. They had faith that they could be healed of their condition, and/or they had confidence in his ability to help them become healed.

A mental attitude that reflects spiritual values is a positive first step toward being healed. Cayce put it this way: *"The closer the body will keep to the truths and the dependence on the abilities latent within self through trust in spiritual things, the quicker will be the response in the physical body. For all healing, mental or material, is attuning each atom of the body, each reflex of the brain forces, to the awareness of the Divine that lies within each atom, each cell of the body."* (3384-2)

It is possible that a change in attitudes may heal a physical problem even before the malady is detected. This happened to one of the most remarkable people I've had the privilege of knowing.

In 1962 I moved to Washington State to enroll in college. For four months prior to college I worked in Seattle and lived in a boarding house. It was owned and operated by lady while the tenants and her three employees were all males. We tenants were a diverse group of six to eight men who worked in various occupations.

Mrs. Jensen, the landlady, had a unique staff. Brady, the cook, was a former lumberjack, roughhewn and course-voiced, who had major physical problems, including a brain tumor which he was unaware of, according to Mrs. Jensen. He moved slowly and had difficulty breathing as he went about his cooking.

Housekeeping and miscellaneous chores around the house were done by the other two male employees. One, with a ready laugh and seemingly above-average intelligence, was, however, emotionally immature and would have difficulty holding a job elsewhere. The other appeared to have little interest or energy for his duties but, nonetheless, managed to keep his job.

Mrs. Jensen was a short, thin woman, under five feet, with bowed legs which caused her to sway from side to side as she walked. She had a breathing problem and made a wheezing sound yet voiced no complaints about her condition. Indeed, she often went to Brady's rescue when he lost his breath climbing chairs or from some other strenuous effort. Once I heard him call for her help late at night. She came as fast as she could with a bit of brandy which she said helped him recover his breath.

While she was not one to talk about spiritual values, Mrs. Jensen obviously was more concerned about the well-being of others than her own problems. She ran the boarding house with three employees who depended on her more than she did on them. She put up with the roughness of the paying tenants without letting them get out of hand. But she was certainly no pushover. She was straightforward and unpretentious, and had a great sense of humor. As best I can remember she never once criticized or preached to any of us. Still, every Sunday she dressed up in fine clothes and a hat and went off to church with her lady friends.

Mrs. Jensen was in her late 70s if not older. Most people in her condition and at her age would be cared for by their families or would be in a nursing home. I have seen people in nursing homes that were in better physical condition than she. But I have seen no one in a nursing home with her spirit and self-reliance.

That was the real miracle of Mrs. Jensen – her attitude. She told me that some years before she had changed her way of thinking and thus her lifestyle. She didn't go into detail except to say that for one thing she had decided to stop worrying. She said that sometimes after she had changed her thinking she went to a doctor for a checkup. He discovered she had scars where stomach ulcers had been. She had not known she had ulcers so she'd had no treatment for them. They had healed spontaneously.

The way Mrs. Jensen related her story without making any connection between a change in attitude and the ulcers healing, left me to figure it out it. It did not impress me at the time. Only years later when I became interested in healing did I realize what she had told me. Her attitude, indeed her whole unselfish lifestyle, was a testimony of spiritual values not preached but lived, and of the sustaining and healing influence of thought upon life.

Mrs. Jensen seems to exemplify the kind of life Edgar Cayce was talking about in this reading:

... as the body may dedicate its life and its abilities to a definite service, to the creative forces or God, there will be healing forces brought to the body. This requires then that the mental attitude be such as to not only proclaim or announce a belief in the Divine, and a promise to dedicate itself to same, but the entity must <u>consistently</u> live such. (3121-1)

The effect of attitudes and emotions on health is not a recent revelation. The fruits of the spirit, the Golden rule, and unselfish thoughts and actions foster health and healing. Positive and constructive attitudes are life-supporting. Negative attitudes such as hate, fear, worry, ill-will, and a refusal to forgive others and ourselves, take their toll on our physical as well as mental well-being.

Cayce often emphasized the mind-body connection. Anger, he said in reading number 3510-1, *"...can destroy the brain as well as any disease. For it is itself a disease of the mind."*

There is no more direct reference as to the affect of mental attitude on physical health than stated in the fifth book of the Old Testament: *"... I have set before you life and death, blessing and cursing; therefore choose life."* (Deut. 30:19)

When physical or mental challenges present themselves, it is then that we need more than ever to focus on spiritual, constructive attitudes. And that can be a formidable task. We are required to become more loving, more unselfish, at a time when an aliment draws our attention to ourselves. When pain and illness dominate our experience, fear and doubt often accompany them. But faith and the right attitude can overcome fear. And faith can be increased and fortified by renewing or improving our relationship with God.

"Then, the healing may come through the attitude of the body-mind to Creative Forces, as it applies to its relationships to others," Cayce advised in reading 2990-1.

The Bible assures us that God, the Creative Forces, cares and will respond if we seek His help: *"when you call I will answer and answer speedily."* (Ps. 102:2) This not only applies to our quest for physical healing, but also for the healing of destructive habits.

In healing ourselves of unhealthy habits, if we can substitute something more desirable, or at least equally desirable, we may be more likely to break a habit. For example, a habit such as snacking on candy may be overcome by substituting more healthy snacks such as fruit. We can get additional help from our subconscious mind by visualizing eating fruit and by imagining its taste. But first there must be the sincere desire to overcome the habit. And this desire to end the habit must, of course, be greater than the desire to continue it. Even if we know that a habit is bad for as, without the desire for change the habit will continue.

"Would you be healed?" Christ asked the crippled man at a pool where the first person into the water, after an angel stirred it, would be healed. But, because of his handicap, each time the angel came and stirred the pool, someone else would get into it before the man could reach it. He wanted to be the first there, he desired to be healed, but he was not fast enough and had no one to help him get to the pool. He explained the situation to Jesus and Christ healed him.

Sometimes if our desire to be healed is strong enough, help will come in unexpected ways. From personal experience I know that this can happen. I believe it was a form of spiritual healing—albeit an unusual one—which cured me of the cigarette smoking habit. Actually, I quit smoking twice. The first time, however, proved not to be permanent. That time I quit out of fear. The second time was what I consider to be a spiritual healing experience.

The first time I quit I had been smoking about eight years. I had just moved to take a new job in another city, had a temporary apartment, and a few days to orient myself to my new surroundings. Both the job and the unfamiliar environment caused me some apprehension, and I found myself smoking even more than usual. That brought on pains in my chest which scared me so badly that I quit smoking. It wasn't easy to quit. The desire for cigarettes remained with me for several years.

After about five years later, in 1970, I began another job. During those five years I had not smoked even once. I thought I had overcome the habit. Not so! After a few months on this new job, I got the notion to have a cigarette with the arrogant assumption that it was okay to give in to my whim because I had beat the habit. Much to my dismay, within no time I was hooked again. I fought it. But it was a losing battle.

Out of frustration I begin saying short prayers at odd times during the day. These prayers were simple "quickies," such as, "Lord, help me stop this smoking!" They were said unceremoniously, on the spur of the moment, any time I thought of doing them. They were not, however, done repetitiously, nor were they said every day. But they were said with sincerity and emotion.

Smoking had a noticeable effect on my body. At the inhaling of smoke from my first cigarette of the day, I could feel what seemed like a sluggishness seeping into my arteries, down my arms and legs, and also into my head. It felt as though the smoke itself slowly moved from my lungs throughout my whole circulatory system. I definitely did not like what this habit was doing to my physical body.

Neither did I enjoy smoking. It left a bad taste in my mouth which greeted me the first thing in the morning. It permeated not only my clothes with the smell of tobacco smoke, but also my paperwork on my job. The latter was not obvious to me, but it was to others. Once, my supervisor had taken some of my work home with him to proofread. He and his wife detected a smell of cigarette smoke, but they did not smoke and did not at first know the origin of the smell. Then they noticed it was coming from my paperwork that my boss was reading. I was so used to the smell of smoke that I was not aware that it saturated even my papers.

I came to hate smoking and the hold it had over me. Many times I switched cigarette brands trying to find one that I liked without success. Eventually my thoughts, feelings, and prayers must have tipped the scales in favor of healing. For in December 1973 I had an experience which cured me of the smoking habit once and for all. It was a singular occurrence, very unpleasant, and powerful enough to rid my body and mind of the need and desire for tobacco.

One night after going out for a spaghetti dinner, I found myself at three in the morning in bed, wide awake, smoking, and feeling terrible. Whether I said my usual, "Lord, help me break the cigarette habit," or if I berated myself for smoking, I do not recall. But I will never forget what happened next. I suddenly got sick and begin to vomit. My upset stomach continued off and on over a six-hour period during which time my body threw up what I believe to be tobacco residue which my system had accumulated over the years. It was the worst upset stomach I ever had.

When my nausea finally ended, I discovered cigarettes had completely lost their appeal to me. I had no desire for them whatsoever. Indeed, I could not even stand to be within smelling range of cigarette smoke. And it remains a mystery to me that even now over forty years later, my aversion to tobacco smoke remains as strong as ever.

At first analysis there seems to be little in my attitudes and actions that could have brought about such a sudden and dramatic cure. However, in light of what I know now, there were at least two factors working in my favor. First was my ongoing praying for relief from the habit. Second was my sincere desire to quit. There was nothing about smoking that appealed to me anymore; it had become just a nervous habit. There is no doubt in my mind that prayer and desire triggered the experience which cured me of the habit. This is just an example of one of the many unpredictable ways that spiritual healing can occur.

Cayce's Perspective on Spiritual Healing

The Edgar Cayce trance readings present a unique view of spiritual healing which not only solves some of the mystery surrounding the subject, but in so doing gives us a better understanding of God's relationship to human-kind.

Cayce gave a number of psychic readings solely to explain the process of spiritual healing. The reading quoted below gives insights that do much to remove the mystery of healing:

[The conductor to Mr. Cayce]: You will have before you the laws of spiritual healing. You will give a discourse at this time on psychic (spiritual) healing, describing just what takes place in the body and mind of one healed...

EC: Yes, we have the laws that govern spiritual or psychic healing. Much has been given through these channels from time to time respecting that necessary in the individual experience for healing.

As we have indicated, the body-physical is an atomic structure subject to the laws of its environment, its heredity, its soul development.

The activity, then, is to create or make a balance in the necessary units of the influence or force that is set in motion as the body in the material form, through the motivating force of spiritual activity, sets in motion.

It is seen that each atom, each corpuscle, has within same the whole form of the universe—within its <u>own</u> structure.

As for the physical body, this is made up of the elements of the various natures that keep same in its motion necessary for sustaining its equilibrium; as begun from its (the individual body's) first cause.

If in the atomic forces there becomes an over-balancing, and injury, a happening, an accident, there are certain atomic forces destroyed or others increased; that to the physical body become either such as to add to or take from the "elan vital" [or creative energy] that makes for the motivating forces through that particular or individual activity.

Then, in meeting these it becomes necessary for the creating of that influence within each individual body to bring a balance necessary for its continued activity about each of the atomic centers its own rotary or creative force, its own elements for the ability of resuscitating, revivifying, such influence or force in the body.

How then, does the activity of any influence act upon the individual system for bringing <u>healing</u> in the wake or the consciousness, to become conscious of its desire?

When a body, separate from that one ill, then, has so attuned or raised its own vibrations sufficiently, it may – by the motion of the spoken word – awaken the activity of the emotions to such an extent as to revivify, resuscitate or to change the rotary force or influence or the atomic forces in the activity of the structural portion, or the <u>vital</u> forces of a body, in such a way and manner as to set it again in motion.

Thus does spiritual or psychic influence of body upon body bring healing to any individual; where another body may raise that necessary influence in the hormone of the circulatory forces as to take from that within itself to revivify or resuscitate diseased, disordered or distressed conditions within a body.

For, as has been said oft, any manner in which healing comes—whether by the laying on of hands, prayer, by a look, by the application of any mechanical influence or any of those forces in materia medica – must be of such a nature as to produce that necessary within those forces about the atomic centers of a given body for it to bring resuscitating or healing. 281-24

We can better understand why spiritual healing, indeed, healing from any source, involves the very atoms of the body as Cayce takes us one step further and explains God's manifestation in humankind at the physical level.

... see, feel, know—as [various treatments] *are being made – that these channels and measures through which the Divine may operate for effective activity in the body.*

And as the electrical vibrations are given, know that life itself—to be sure—is the creative forces or God, yet in its manifestation in man are electrical or vibratory.

Know then that the force in nature that is called electrical or electricity is at same force ye worship as Creative or God in action!

Seeing this, feeling this, knowing this, ye will find that not only does the body become revivified, but by the creating in every atom of its being the knowledge of the activity of this creative force or principal as related to spirit, mind, body – all three are renewed. For these are as the trinity in the body, these are as the trinity in the principles of the very life force itself – as the Father, the Son, the Spirit—the body, divine, the spirit—these are one. One Spirit, one God, one activity. Then see Him, know Him, in those influences. For even as the Son gave,

"I of myself may do nothing, but as the Father working in me, through me." (1299-1)

Because electricity plays a role in almost every aspect of modern life, it is difficult to comprehend how this same energy can be a manifestation of God. In other Cayce readings he makes a distinction between two kinds of vibration, or electricity. In a reading 1861-16, he gave that, *"Life in its manifestation is vibration. Electricity is vibration. But vibration that is creative is one thing. Vibration that is destructive is another. Yet they may be from the same source."* Cayce further clarifies the concept in reading 2828-4: *"Electricity or vibration is that same energy same power, ye call God. Not that God is an electric light or an electric machine, but that vibration that is creative is of that same energy as life itself."*

These insights into the nature of God help us understand how we can facilitate healing. If we are able to raise our vibrations to a level that is creative, and then send these by prayer, thought, word, or touch to another, they have the ability to temporarily raise the vibrations in another. When we raise our vibrations, which Cayce says are electrical, we see that our thoughts then produce this creative electrical energy. What we transmit in our prayers, thoughts, or healing touch is an actual energy. This energy, directed by the intention of the sender, or healer, reaches and influences vibrations of the recipient at the level of atoms and molecules. The raised vibrations –creative electrical energy—influences the electrical energy in its intended receiver, when that person is in agreement with or receptive to such vibrations.

That thoughts are actual things is hard to comprehend. But if we can accept this as true, then we can better accept the idea that they can have an effect on the object which receives them.

The unseen force of the vibrations we send forth for healing accomplishes its purpose according to the sincerity, intention, and focus or direction of the energy.

The word "vibration" was a household word in the 1960s. Its meaning then was practically the same as our use of it here except we learn from the Cayce readings of its more far-reaching and purposeful employment. We used to say a person had good or bad "vibes," meaning that it was either pleasant or unpleasant to be around that person. And though the term "vibes" is no longer widely used, we can still feel when a person makes us uncomfortable, or if we like to be with him or her. It has always been this way. This is because we send out positive or negative vibrations from our attitude, thoughts, and state of mind. We are always thinking when we're awake. And this thinking always sends out electrical vibrations. Sometimes our thoughts are not so strong as to transmit noticeable vibrations. Other times they are so forceful, either in a positive or negative way that they can be physically felt by others.

It is this same vibratory force that we are able to raise for the purpose of healing. And it is the same vibratory force that Jesus radiated. The main difference between our thinking and the consciousness of Christ is that He sustained vibrations at the creative or healing level, whereas we have to make a special effort to raise our vibrations to His level, and then we usually can do so only for very short periods of time. But in these short periods of time we are privileged to participate, to facilitate healings.

The Healings of Jesus

To say that Jesus had "good vibes" sounds almost irreverent. But if we accept the proposition as fact that he was God incarnate, and that God is the highest vibration – the creative force of the universe—then Jesus, being synonymous in consciousness with God, has that same highest vibration possible. Then to say that Jesus had good vibes is not irreverent; it is a gross understatement. He went about teaching what humanity had never heard before and healing as none before him.

That Christ radiated healing energy was evidenced by the occasions when people were healed by merely touching his clothes. The incident in the Bible in which a woman touched his garment, knowing that if she did so she would be healed, is only one of many such healings he did. In Matthew we read that Christ healed a large number of people in this way:

... they came into the land of Gennesaret. And when the man of that place had knowledge of Jesus, they sent out into all that country round about, and brought unto him all that were diseased. And besought him that they might only touch the hem of his garment: and as many as touched were made perfectly whole. (Matt. 14:34-36)

Of all the hundreds, perhaps thousands, of people Jesus healed, only a few are discussed in any detail in the Bible. And a number of these are repeated in the Gospels. Accounts of his healings, which are repeated with only minor differences in details, appear to be unnecessary. For example the case mentioned above of the woman touching his garment in order to be healed is not only in Matthew (9:18-24), but also in Mark (5:25-34), and in Luke (8:43-48). We do know that the four Gospels were written at different times and for different peoples. Biblical scholars tell us that Matthew wrote for the Jews, Mark wrote for the Romans, and Luke for the Greeks, while John wrote for the spiritual needs of all humankind. How and why they came to choose the same healings to write about is a matter of conjecture.

However, if we study these we find they emphasize certain aspects of Jesus' approach to healing. Possibly they were selected because they best illustrate his methods. And that they were given to us not just as a historical record, but that we may learn from them. While Jesus did not seem to seek out people to heal, neither did He turn anyone away. It is certainly possible that He did go out of his way to offer healing to the sick who could not come to Him. This was evidenced in the incident previously cited when Christ went out of His way to heal the crippled man who could not get to the healing pool. But usually he was thronged by people coming to Him for healing.

Jesus never required anyone to justify being healed. He told no one that he or she did not deserve to be healed. He healed everyone without regard as to the type of illness, status in society, or moral behavior. People did have to qualify for healing, however. But those qualifications were mental attributes or requirements which had nothing to do with morals, or social standing, or the illness.

Two things were required of those who sought healing from Jesus: the desire to be healed and belief that he could heal them.

Contrary to what we would like to think, not all of us sincerely desire to be healed of all our ailments. That is not to say that we want to be sick or to have some other form of physical or mental difficulty. Yet, often we will not pay the price of healing in terms of our willingness to do our share to regain and maintain health. Lack of desire for healing is reflected in something as simple as refusing to seek or accept medical help for an ailment, or being unwilling to change an attitude responsible for an illness. And though Jesus never turned anyone away who asked Him for healing, he did in some cases tell the healed person to, *"Go and sin no more least a worst fate befall you."* (John 5:14)

So Jesus healed all who desired it from Him. But unless they desire to stay well, with the willingness to change the attitudes or actions responsible for their affliction, Jesus' healings would be only temporary. When one desires to be healed to the extent of doing what is required to get well and stay well, he or she is not only likely to find healing, but will most likely experience great spiritual growth in the process. For in the last analysis, true healing is spiritual and not simply a physical cure.

Belief is the foundation of spiritual healing. As great a healer as Christ was, He could not heal those who had no faith in His ability to do so. Those who did not believe in His teaching, or in who He was, did not have confidence in Him. They doubted, or chose not to believe.

"But though he had done so many miracles before them, yet they believed not on him... He hath blinded their eyes, and hardened their heart; that they should not see with their eyes, nor understand with their heart, and be converted, and I should heal them." (John 12:37, 40)

For those who desired to be healed and believed Jesus could heal them, He usually employed just two methods: the spoken word and touch. Most often He used the spoken word. And when He used touch to heal, the spoken word usually accompanied his touch.

Sometimes Jesus asked the afflicted what they desired of him. If they replied that they wanted to be healed, it was typical of Jesus to ask if they believed He was able to heal them. After they had expressed both their desire to be healed and affirmed their belief that He could heal them, His usual response was similar to, *"Your faith has made you whole."* (Mark 5:34) Sometimes He instructed the healed person to do something, such as show himself to a priest after being healed.

Matthew 9:27-30 is an excellent example of Jesus' usual method of healing:

And when Jesus departed thence [after raising Jairus's daughter], two blind men followed him, crying, and saying, "Thou son of David, have mercy on us."

And when he was come into the house, two blind men came to him: and Jesus saith unto them, "Believe ye that I am able to do this?" They said unto him, "Yea, Lord."

Then he touched their eyes, saying, "According to your faith be it unto you."

And their eyes were opened; and Jesus strictly charged them, saying, "See that no man know it."

The simplicity of his methods is deceiving. Jesus was a man of great understanding and compassion. His understanding of human nature and human potential gave Him the wisdom to deal with any physical or mental illness. His oneness with God's plan for human redemption and God's creative, healing nature, gave him the compassion and ability to heal. With this knowledge he not only knew how to heal, but why he could heal. He didn't just believe he could heal, he *knew* he could. Nonetheless, without belief on the part of those sick he could not or would not heal them.

Suggestive Magnetic Therapy and Faith Healing

There are significant differences in "faith healing" and the practice of suggestive magnetic therapy, though both are forms of spiritual healing.

Faith healing seeks instantaneous results and usually calls upon God and/or an omnipresent Jesus to heal. The healer uses both touch and speech in a typical healing session. Such sessions can take less than a minute. And they are not usually repeated, the healer relying on the one attempt only. If the one session doesn't accomplish healing, more sessions are not usually offered. Faith healing relies totally on belief as the name implies. Healing, when it happens, is spontaneous, the self-healing mechanism of the body responded to divine intervention (or raised vibrations) facilitated by the healer with the cooperation of the person seeking to be healed.

Permanence of such healing – as with healing from any source—depends upon the person healed. If one eliminates from one's life, the cause of the ailment, it is not likely to return. If the cause is not eliminated, a relapse or worse may occur.

Faith healing is usually done in churches or evangelical meetings and can have a few people to thousands in attendance.

In contrast, suggestive magnetic therapy is done in private, the facilitator and subject usually should be the only ones present. Reason for this is that the facilitator must be able to concentrate on what he or she is doing, and the subject must remain in a relaxed, passive state of consciousness. With others in attendance, the facilitator and the subject face possible distractions and skepticism. Either can prohibit whatever success the therapy might otherwise garner. On the other hand, there may be in attendance a few family members or friends of the ailing person if they are in perfect agreement with the therapy and wish to lend spiritual support. Such support in this case is best provided by having those present meditating on one specific affirmation. More will be said about this in Chapter 5.

Being a spiritual healing art and not a science, suggestive magnetic therapy does not take a predetermined number of sessions to accomplish healing. There are just too many variables. Healing depends on both facilitator and subject. It is the state of consciousness of both that invites or allows God, the healing vibration, to act within the subject's body to bring about healing. It is the role of the facilitator to prepare the best he or she can to administer the therapy. Likewise, it is the role of the subject to prepare for the session knowing that it is a cooperative effort.

Healing, and the time it takes for healing to happen, also depends on God. Healer and the subject must do all they can, the best they can, and leave the results to God. Whether it takes only one suggestive magnetic therapy session or many, many sessions over a period of weeks, even months or more, to bring about healing, that must not be the concern of those involved. And, as with any healing endeavors, success is not guaranteed.

However, there is one benefit derived from this therapy that seldom results from any other form of healing including faith healing: both patient and healer grow spiritually in the process. The more treatments that are given to any one person, the more likely the participants will feel that the spiritual relationship between them-selves and God is enhanced. Subject and healer will experience a sense of spiritual bonding if the therapy is done correctly. Even if healing is not forthcoming in the physical, there may be great healing on the spiritual level, not just in the unconscious or soul, but also in the conscious mind. This is simply a natural result of the spiritual preparation required to do suggestive magnetic therapy and the action of Spirit in the healing sessions.

Unlike most of the healing methods, the roles of participants in suggestive magnetic therapy are reversible. For example, a family member suffering from an ailment one week and treated by another family member may, at a later date, take on the role of healer for the same person who had facilitated his or her healing sessions previously. It is simply a matter of slightly different preparation for each, but there is a major difference in the activity of each during the session itself. While preparation for both is primarily prayer and meditation, the state of consciousness of the subject during the healing session is passive in contrast to that of the healer which is active.

Suggestive magnetic therapy is based upon the healing methods of Christ. It employs both the voice and touch to facilitate healing. And it requires desire for healing, confidence in the healer, and the belief that healing is possible on the part of the afflicted. The healer must have faith that this particular healing method can reach the Creative Forces within his or her subject to overcome the destructive vibrations causing the illness. The healer's attitude should reflect Jesus' statement that, *"Of myself I can do nothing; it is the father within that does the work."* (John 8:28)

How does one become a healer? Cayce reiterates the process in this reading:

... let's analyze healing for the moment, to those that must consciously...see and reason, see a material demonstration, occasionally at least! Each atomic force of a physical body is made up of its units of positive and

negative forces that bring it into a material plane. These are of the ether, or atomic forces, being electrical in nature as they enter into a material basis, or become matter in its ability to take on or throw off. So as a group [or individual] may raise the atomic vibrations that make for those positive forces as bring divine force and action into a material plane, those that are destructive are broken down by the raising of that vibration! That's material, see? This is done through Creative Forces, which are God in manifestation! Hence, as self brings those little things necessary [preparation, attunement] ...So does the entity become the healer. 281-3

With our conscious minds we create an environment which makes spiritual healing possible. Through the subject's subconscious mind comes the healing response. It is the subconscious with which the Creative Forces interact to change the vibrations within the body. And the motivating force in the conscious mind to which the unconscious responds is desire, supported by belief, the foundation of all spiritual healing.

3

THE SUBCONSCIOUS AND HEALING

The importance of belief in healing was emphasized in the last chapter. Indeed, even Jesus did not heal those who lacked faith. Belief is *the* prerequisite to spiritual healing. And that is where the subconscious comes into play in the healing process. For it is the subconscious which, acting on belief of the conscious mind, that opens the door to the Divine to overcome destructive forces in the physical body.

Those facilitating suggestive magnetic therapy should prepare for healing sessions by attuning to the Creative Forces, and by being aware that the subconscious mind of the subject must be reached for healing to begin. We are most concerned with the subconscious mind of the person seeking healing, and not that of the healing facilitator, because it is within the subconscious of the ailing person that spontaneous healing is to be prompted.

If we were using "faith healing" there would be no need for this study. That is because faith healing employs no specific techniques, nor does it require understanding of the healing process. On the other hand, suggestive magnetic therapy does employee specific methods. With knowledge of the unconscious the healing facilitator does not rely solely on faith, but also on his understanding of how and why the subconscious functions in the spiritual healing process.

Edgar Cayce's Concept of the Unconscious

Cayce's perspective from the trance state gave him a unique panorama of the subconscious and its relationship with other "hidden" aspects of humankind—the soul, superconscious, and spirit:

[Mind] is the active force in an animate object; that is the spark, or the image of the Maker. Mind is the factor that is in direct opposition of will. Mind being that control of, or being the spark of the Maker, the will, the individual when we reach plane of man. Mind being and is the factor governing the contention, or the interlaying space, if you please, between the physical to the soul, and the soul to the spirit forces within the individual or animate forces...Mind is that that reasons the impressions from the senses, as they manifest before the individual. 3744-2

Cayce distinguishes between what he calls the super-conscious and the subconscious minds. The subcon-scious controls the physical body and resides between the soul and the body, while the superconscious occupies an area between the soul and spirit forces. The following readings help to clarify these ideas:

... The mind in the physical body [is] the subconscious, the conscious, through which the entity manifests in the physical world...

The superconscious [is] the divide, that oneness lying between the soul and the spirit force, within the spiritual entity. Not of earth forces at all, only awakened with the spiritual indwelling and acquired individually. 900-21

According to Cayce, when we die we shed the physical body and are then more conscious of the other aspects of ourselves:

When the body physical lays aside the material body, that in the physical called soul becomes the body of the entity, and that called the superconscious the consciousness of the entity, as the subconscious is to the physical body. The subconscious [is] the mind or intellect of the body.(900-304)

Cayce appears to be saying here that both our objective conscious mind and the subjective subconscious mind comprise our consciousness when we are alive here on earth. Then when we die what is now our soul and subconscious in the earth plane becomes our body and our awareness. And what is now our superconscious mind then becomes our subconscious. The diagram on the next page illustrates the relationships between the various levels of the unconscious, the conscious mind, and both our physical and soul bodies.

Amenability of the subconscious

Our subconscious mind is inextricably woven into the physical body we inhabit. Not only is it involved in what we call consciousness—presenting us with dreams and

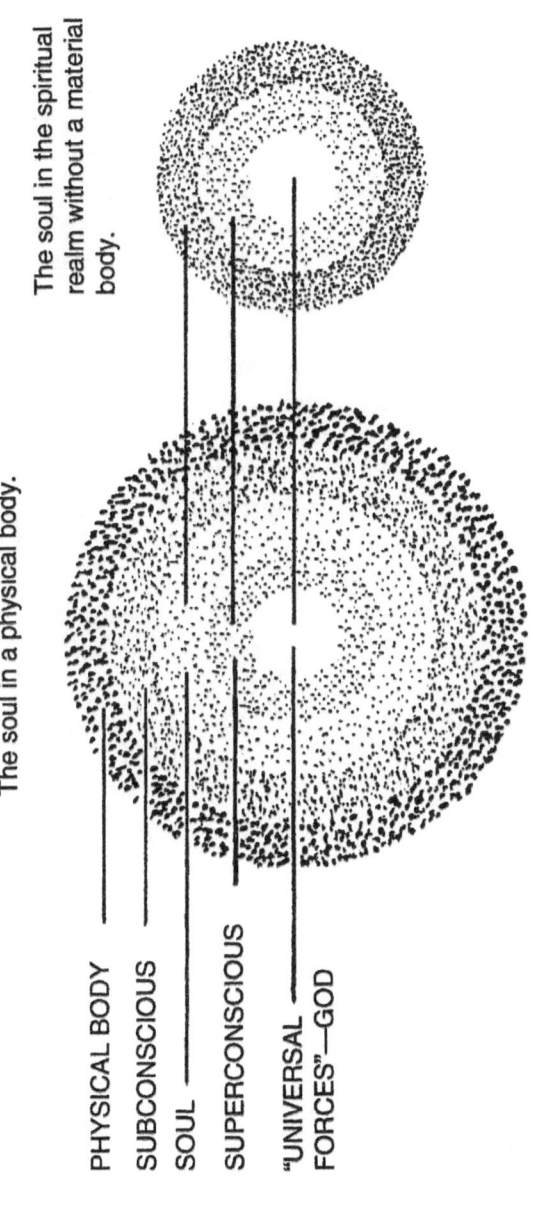

The soul in a physical body.

The soul in the spiritual realm without a material body.

PHYSICAL BODY

SUBCONSCIOUS

SOUL

SUPERCONSCIOUS

"UNIVERSAL FORCES"—GOD

"When the body physical lays aside the material body, that in the physical called soul becomes the body of the entity, and that called the superconscious [becomes] the consciousness of the entity, as the subconscious is to the physical body." (900-304) other messages—it also oversees the operations of the physical body. Often our subconscious warns us of problems within the body through dreams. Consciousness, especially the subconscious, may be embedded in the physical fabric of our being at the atomic level. Cayce mentions the "mind of the atom." Scientists tell us that atoms somehow communicate. Can it be that this intelligent life force we call God permeates our physical body? According to Cayce that is exactly the case. For every atom, every cell is alive because of the electrical vibrations that sustain them.

These very same vibrations that maintain life often go awry. They can become disoriented or have their vibrations change to those that result in disease. They may do this whenever attitudes, emotions, or beliefs are contrary to supporting life. By the same token, a change in consciousness can change our vibrations back to life-supporting ones. *"I have set before you this day life and death, blessing and cursing, choose thou"* (Deut. 30:19)

That both the unconscious, with all its wisdom, and the physical body, with this tremendous complexity, can be influenced by the conscious mind seems unlikely. It is as if the captain of the ship is the least qualified to direct it. Yet, that is the situation. The subconscious is subject to the activities of the conscious mind. We could say it is the servant of the conscious mind.

The subconscious mind won't argue with the messages sent to it. It simply records the messages and often acts upon them, but it does not censor them. It follows directions from the conscious mind. When there are no new directions, no new beliefs, it follows previous beliefs as habit.

Wouldn't it be convenient if our unconscious would filter out unhealthy thoughts sent to it? Then we would not need to be concerned with the consequences of our attitudes on our physical well-being. We would not be accountable because unhealthy thoughts simply would not reach the subconscious. But, alas, such is not the case; we create our own destiny by choices made at the conscious level—"free will" it's called. And while the subconscious will not weed out unhealthy thoughts, we do get feedback. Warnings come to us from the unconscious which, if not heeded, may result in illness or disease.

We know that habits are formed by repetition at the conscious level that take hold in the subconscious. Habits are difficult to break for this very reason. To loosen them, to free ourselves, it requires uprooting them. This not only refers to habits such as smoking, but it also applies to thinking habits and beliefs which may lead to physical problems. If we change what we continually feed into our subconscious, it will respond accordingly. The subconscious has no choice. Choice is a function of the conscious mind: *"... each soul, each mind, each entity is endowed with its choice. And the choice is a result of the application of self in its relationships to that which is its ideal – and finds manifestation in what individuals call habit, or subconscious activity. Yet it has its inception in that of choice."* (830-2)

The Subconscious Controls the Physical Body

Edgar Cayce diagnosed his own physical problems while in a trance state of consciousness. To resolve some of these problems he could tell the conductor of the reading what suggestions he should be given.

It's interesting to note that he could not give himself the suggestion while in trance. Though he knew in his subconscious state what needed to be said to him while in that state, it required another person to repeat a suggestion to him. This fact emphasizes the point that the subconscious cannot direct itself.

Implementing directions from the conscious mind – its own conscious mind or from another—even to change conditions in the physical body is, however one of the subconscious mind's faculties. Cayce reading number 294-11 supports this claim.

To give that necessary then for this body [Edgar Cayce], in the present condition, give those suggestions, for the body in this psychic condition is amenable to suggestion. Relieve then through increased circulation to those parts that do not vibrate properly, and removing the dross from those conditions the vibration will come the normal condition in the body... Do that.

[Conductor]: *Now the circulation will increase to the parts that need be, so that it will remove the trouble with the speech and the rest of the body that needs it. When it has been relieved, you will say, "This trouble is re-moved." When the trouble is removed the circulation will become normal in the body again.*

[Cayce's reply, still in trance]: *It is removed.*

Gladys Davis, Cayce's stenographer who was present at practically all of his trance readings after 1923, verified the effectiveness of the suggestion given Cayce. She noted that whenever Cayce lost his voice because of physical or mental strain the problem would be resolved simply by giving him the above suggestion while he was in trance. Gladys reported that many times she witnessed the color return to his face and throat as a circulation returned to normal after the above suggestion was given.

The human body is an unbelievably complex system requiring a super intelligence to oversee and regulate it.

That the subconscious does this job appears to be true. *"The subconscious [is] the superconscious of the physical entity, partaking then of the soul forces and of the material plane..."* (900-31) We can more fully appreciate Cayce's statement that the subconscious is the "superconscious" at the physical body when we consider the amazing complexity of the body.

Trillions of living cells cooperating with each other form a body—every cell composed of many atoms, each a universe unto itself, active, vibrating—electrical. Atoms, molecules, cells, vibrating with life, electricity, come together to form the different components of a physical body. It is mind-boggling.

In the larger picture, the communication, the interaction necessary among the body's various structures, processes, organs, nerves, and fluids make it a smoothly operating unit.

Sensory messages create our awareness of the world outside our body and in some cases within our body. Internal messages relay to the brain activities within the body, constantly monitoring, coordinating, and regulating the functioning and processes within the body. These messages, both sensory and internal, are received by the nerves and transmitted as electrical impulses to the brain for processing. The brain, a tremendous electro-magnetic organ, is a laboratory of the subconscious, translating, analyzing, processing, and responding to sensory and internal messages.

All this activity necessary to sustain our physical bodies is performed without conscious direction or effort on our part. It is done below the conscious mind, under control of the subconscious mind. Usually we do not consciously get involved with the internal workings of our body. Yet we do affect it with our thoughts, attitudes, and emotions. Orthodox medicine acknowledges this to a degree. And many medical professionals also acknowledge that conscious mental and spiritual activities such as positive thinking, prayer, and meditation, affect the body even to the point of healing it. But the belief that the subconscious mind controls the internal activities of the body would no doubt be scoffed at by most in the medical professions.

However, this idea is not new. During the last century and even before that, it was accepted as fact by those who practiced suggestive therapeutics, mental therapeutics, magnetic healing, mesmerism, and other similar healing arts. It is also part of the New Thought philosophy and that of the founders of Unity, Religious Science, and Christian Science.

In his remarkable book, *The Law of Psychic Phenomenon*, Thomson J. Hudson succinctly states the basis of this belief:

... The fundamental principles which lie at the foundation of mental therapeutics [are] –
1. The subjective [subconscious] mind exercises complete control over the functions and sensations of the body.
2. The subjective mind is constantly amenable to control by the suggestions of the objective mind.
3. These two propositions being true, the conclusion is obvious, that the functions and sensations of the body can be controlled by suggestions of the objective mind.

What Heals, God or the Subconscious?

We are now left with this obvious question: Is it the subconscious mind that does the healing or is it God, the Universal Creative Energy that heals? This is a legitimate question, for if it is the subconscious that heals, why even bring God into the picture? Why not just leave God out altogether and deal solely with the subconscious without any spiritual overtones?

Actually, no reference to spirituality is required in the practice of suggestion or magnetic healing with the hands. A person may use these methods with success without any belief in a Creator. However, it is not wise to do so unless such a person's intentions and attitudes are constructive and unselfish.

The safest route to take in facilitating healing is to do so within a spiritual context and environment. Otherwise the healer is on his or her own to cope with the negative influences that could eventually lead to mental, emotional, or physical health problems in the healer. Temptation can be strong to put oneself on a pedestal as being a *healer*. However, if one acknowledges that he or she is only instrumental in helping the healing process, then one is much more likely to avoid having to deal with negative influences that could arise.

Yes, healing can happen simply by addressing the subconscious with suggestions that instill belief. However to do suggestive magnetic therapy within a spiritual framework not only ensures a safe environment, but rewards the facilitator with an indefinable appreciation of the Creator, and an inner spiritual connection with those that person has the privilege to help.

While one might take the position that spirituality is not a factor in healing, Cayce's readings tell us that God does in fact do the healing. With our definition of God expanded to include life itself, or the creative force of the universe, we have little difficulty in understanding or accepting Cayce's explanations. The following reading tells us how God, or the "Universal Forces," and the subconscious both are involved in the healing process:

The superconscious mind [is] that of the spiritual entity, and in action only when the subconscious is become the conscious mind...through the superconscious the Universal Forces are made active in subconsciousness. (900-31)

An interpretation of this reading is illustrated in diagram form below.

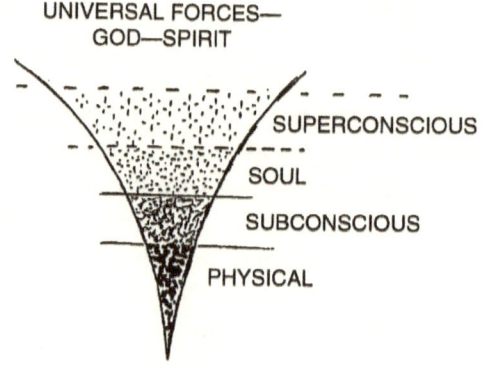

UNIVERSAL FORCES—
GOD—SPIRIT

SUPERCONSCIOUS

SOUL

SUBCONSCIOUS

PHYSICAL

"I stand at the door and knock . . . "

UNIVERSAL FORCES

SUPERCONSCIOUS

" . . .through
the super-
conscious
the Universal
Forces are made
active in subcon-
sciousness."
(900-31)

SOUL

SUBCONSCIOUS

PHYSICAL

When the Universal forces are made active in the subconscious healing can take place. The subconscious, whose job it is to regulate the *"functions and sensations of the body,"* as Hudson stated, receives help, as it were, from these Universal Forces when disease or illness proves too much for the body to overcome without help. As previously discussed, the body already has its own innate healing ability. But when this built-in ability is overwhelmed by disease and destructive vibrations have the upper hand, the Creative Forces can be petitioned for healing.

In suggestive magnetic therapy, belief, in the form of suggestion, opens the door of the subconscious allowing the Universal Forces to flow through the superconscious into the subconscious. *"I stand at the door and knock, if anyone should open, I will come in and sup with him."* (Rev. 3:20) This universal healing vibration is ever ready to enter if we open the door of our unconscious. If we provide the necessary environment in which healing can happen, it will happen.

Life, being God manifesting at the physical level, permeates our body as electrical energy, vibrations. Our thoughts and actions affect these vibrations either by being in harmony with life or being out of harmony. If the latter occurs, our vibrations become other than creative and illness in some form may ensue.

Healing then involves changing conscious attitudes and beliefs to constructive ones. However, rather than changing our consciousness, we usually seek outside help from traditional or alternative medicine, or spiritual healing. Any or all of these healing efforts can act upon our subconscious to reinstate the creative vibration, resulting in health. However for healing to be permanent, the cause of the disharmony must be eliminated and replaced with life-sustaining attitudes and emotions.

Seldom does the true cause become known. Yet in seeking healing through spiritual avenues we may resolve the cause during the healing process. True healing occurs with a change in the consciousness at a level that gets to the root of the problem. Otherwise, our ailment may only be temporarily alleviated rather than healed, thus only postponing the problem instead of resolving it.

Avenues to the Unconscious

There are many ways the subconscious can be approached for healing purposes. This is achieved with a person in either the normal waking state or in passive states of consciousness.

In the waking state a person's everyday thoughts and experiences reach his or her subconscious where they are recorded as memory. These are not normally intended to have any specific effect upon the subconscious. However, other conscious thoughts and mental activities can influence the subconscious and are intended to do so. Two of the more popular conscious approaches are the use of affirmations and visualization.

Affirmations are short positive statements repeated to oneself. Often they are said at designated times, such as upon rising in the morning and when retiring for the night. The purpose of affirmations is to impress the subconscious by repetition of the statements. They can be said either aloud or mentally to oneself. Affirmations are widely used in New Thought religions such as Religious Science and Unity.

Visualization involves the mental picturing of something one wants to accomplish or to have happen. For example, a basketball player might picture in his mind that he is scoring goals. He simply repeats the scene over and over mentally.

In a college experiment this method proved almost as effective as real-life practice. One group of players actually practiced shooting basketballs an hour each day for a month. Another group practiced only in their imagination by visualizing scoring baskets an hour each day for a month. At the end the month both groups were tested for improvement in their actual basketball shooting skills. The accuracy of the group that had practiced shooting improved twenty-four percent while the group which "practiced" using only visualization improved an impressive twenty-three percent. A third group which did not practice at all showed no increase in their accuracy. This experiment demonstrated what many believe to be true—that *the subconscious mind cannot tell the difference between what is actual and what is imagined!* Visualization is enhanced by including emotions and details in the visualization practice. We will discuss visualization again later.

The passive/receptive states of consciousness in which the subconscious can be assessed may be divided into two areas: those states that can be induced by oneself and those that require another person as facilitator. Meditation, self-hypnosis, and pre-sleep suggestion are examples of self induced states.

Many meditation techniques exist. True meditation is listening to the Divine within. In two of the more widely used techniques in our culture, affirmations and mantras (sounds) are focused upon to the exclusion of other thoughts until the mind is stilled. *"Be still and know that I am God"* is a biblical reference to meditation. Meditation allows us fleeting glimpses of the Divine, not through thought, but with the absence of thought when the conscious mind momentarily rests. This can happen several times during a meditation, or it may not happen at all during a meditation period. It depends on the ability of the meditator to attune to the Divine, the Infinite by bringing his or her mind to a state of peaceful inactivity. It is then that the Universal Forces can become active in the subconscious. Meditation is an important part of preparation for healing and will be discussed in more depth in Chapter 4.

Self-hypnosis, or autosuggestion, involves getting oneself into a passive/receptive mental state. Pre-recorded computer discs are a modern, effective way of doing self- hypnosis. There are commercially produced self-improvement discs sold today. However, one can easily record their own, thus customizing the suggestions for his or her own healing needs.

Pre-sleep and sleep suggestion can also be done with computer discs. Affirmations and visualization can be employed prior to and as one enters the sleep state. The last thoughts and images focused upon as one drifts off into sleep find easy access into the subconscious.

Two passive states of consciousness that can be facilitated by another person include hypnosis and the relaxed state used in suggestive magnetic therapy, which is a lighter passive state then hypnosis.

Hypnosis can range from hardly more than being transfixed in front of a TV, to deep trance states such as Edgar Cayce experienced. Often a licensed hypnotist's practice centers on the resolving of unwanted habits such as smoking. Hypnosis is also effective in blocking pain. It is now used by dentists and some physicians for this purpose. Sidney Weltmer used hypnosis sparingly in his healing work. He preferred to use a lighter passive mental state for his patients because he claimed its results were more permanent.

For our purposes it is this passive state of mind akin to dozing which suggestive magnetic therapy relies on to reach the subconscious mind for healing purposes. To influence the subconscious mind we will use voice, intention, and touch. Of these three, Cayce says that the voice produces the highest vibration. This, however, depends on the individual:

(Q) [404] In the training of the subconscious mind, which is more effective, thought or the spoken word, and why?
(A) *In the training of the subconscious mind, first let it be considered as to <u>what</u> is being acted upon. Then the question will answer itself. The subconscious mind is both consciousness and thought or spirit consciousness. Hence may be best classified, in the physical sense, as a habit. Should such [a person]being acted upon be one that thinks thought would act quicker than the spoken word, then to such [a person] it would! When it is necessary to reach the subconscious of an individual through the senses of the physical <u>body</u>, before it may be visualized by such [a person], then the spoken word would be more effective...Hence that which is spoken (for why the question is asked) to a growing, developing body in oral manner to the sleeping or semi-conscious mind will act the better still! That answers the question for <u>this</u> body!* (262-10)

Singleness of Vision

Because the subconscious does not block input, it is constantly inundated with messages. Much of what comes to the subconscious, while not censored, is not acted upon. When there are conflicting messages at the conscious level, the subconscious naturally gets mixed signals. If the subconscious gets one message it begins to act on, and then receives conflicting messages, they cancel out each other.

Of course, all thoughts and experiences recorded in the subconscious as memory do not change one's consciousness or physical vibrations. Only those thoughts and attitudes that are cemented in the unconscious as belief act to change our physical or conscious selves.

An example of the ineffectiveness of conflicting messages to the subconscious is the often-misunderstood potential of affirmations. A woman recently told me she was using affirmations but without success. She was herself a student of metaphysics and worked in a related profession. She proclaimed, by affirmation, words intended to remedy a problem she had. What she did not realize was that her fears about her situation negated the affirmations. One part of her conscious mind – her emotions – was in conflict with her mental efforts. For as soon as she told me about using the affirmations, she immediately expressed fears about her problem. Fear, as doubt, cancels the good that affirmations might accomplish.

When thoughts and emotions are in agreement, things happen. If positive attitudes and emotions are sustained, healing vibrations result. Unity of conscious activity— singleness of vision—can result in the physical body being full of light, full of the creative vibration. When there is agreement, that is, lack of conflict, the subconscious can respond.

Effective affirmations cannot be at odds with our normal everyday thoughts and feelings. Ideally, affirmations should be a condensation in statement form of our desires and thoughts. It is true that affirmations are used to raise consciousness above ordinary daily thoughts. Nonetheless, until these agree, unless our vision is single, the subconscious is sent conflicting messages.

Suggestions—affirmations used in suggestive magnetic therapy—are a part of the singleness of purpose required to produce a healing environment. Unity of effort of the healing facilitator and the subject are required if healing is to be made possible.

The person seeking to be healed must believe that healing is possible. And the sincere desire to be healed needs to be enhanced by preparing for healing treatments. One also must have a positive attitude toward the healing facilitator and the suggestive magnetic therapy process. On the other hand, the facilitator has to maintain singleness of intention. One's use of hands for healing, and suggestion in the form of affirmations, focuses a single healing purpose. This unity of purpose, thought, and agreement in the consciousness of your subject reaches the subconscious as one single message without conflict. *"If thine eye be single, thy whole body will be for a light."* (Matt. 6:22) It is this biblical truth that suggestive magnetic therapy endeavors to accomplish.

Response Time

Healing takes time. Physical problems are often deep-rooted. Disease is not unlike psychological problems which are not easily resolved. Often they have been a long time developing. Possibly years of mental or physical misuse are the cause of an illness or impairment. Is it any wonder, then, that physical healing also takes time?

The instantaneous healings of Christ and present-day healing miracles are the exception. They do occur. Some are permanent, having eradicated the cause along with the symptom, the ailment itself. The real miracle is elimination of the cause. For without such healing the problem is almost certain to resurface in the same or a completely different symptom. Without getting at the root of a problem it is not truly resolved. That is why Jesus said, *"Go and sin no more lest a worse fate befall you."* (John 5:14)

Fortunate are those whose consciousness is changed by enlightened understanding that results in the formation of new health-sustaining beliefs. The greatest miracle of all is a change in consciousness from old illness-producing attitudes and emotions to new awareness—Christ Consciousness—which is in harmony with life itself.

Yet, we must be patient. The subconscious cannot be pushed or coerced into action. It responds when new belief replaces old. And there is no way of determining the time required for this to happen.

Cayce was frequently asked when a person would be cured of a particular ailment. It was not unusual for him to reply that one should not be concerned about how long it would take. If it were only days, weeks, or even years, those involved should make a commitment to persevere with patience. He told questioners not to begin at all unless willing to continue as long as necessary.

Is it not better for healing to take longer to happen if in so doing it removes the cause of a problem rather than getting a fast cure that may be short-lived? This is not to imply that healings which do occur quickly will not be permanent. On the other hand if healing seems to be taking a long time to occur, it does not mean that nothing is happening at the unconscious level. It does not mean the treatments are not working. One should be content in the possibility that when results take longer it may be because treatments are getting to the source of a deeply rooted problem. And then when healing does happen it may remove more than just the symptom.

There is another positive side to doing many suggestive magnetic treatments for one person. Each treatment session is a spiritual experience. The more opportunities for treating the same person, the more solid becomes a spiritual bonding of those involved. It also brings them in closer contact or harmony with the Creator of life itself. Patience in waiting for a healing response is therefore rewarded in more ways than one.

Many variables determine how long it may take the subconscious to become receptive to healing vibrations. Ability of the healer and subject to provide a healing environment, the depth of the roots of the ailment, and the spiritual lesson to be learned from the problem are all involved.

One of my favorite movies provides an excellent example of the time involved in healing. *Field of Dreams* is a magical movie brimming with supernatural events. In the movie the main character, Ray, has been told by a voice, *"If you build it, they will come."* He is then shown a vision of a baseball field in his cornfield. He does not understand why he is to build the field, but he does it anyway. Neither does he understand who will come once the field is built.

He plows under much of his corn and builds the baseball field seen in his vision. The field is completed but nothing happens. Fall passes, then winter. Still nothing happens. He often gazes out his window at the field with positive expectancy. He knows something is going to happen out there; h e can feel it. Then one night it does. A baseball player appears, and soon after others appear also. Baseball legends, who had long since died, come to play ball. Ray is filled with awe and joy at seeing these players using the field that he and his family have built. However, he does not realize that the question of who will come if the field is built has not yet been answered.

Then one day his father who had been a baseball player in his youth, appears. It is what Ray has waited for without realizing it. After he had built the field that he saw in his vision, it took time for his father to finally appear. When they meet, they are reconciled, healing their broken relationship.

The situation is comparable to the subconscious and the healing process. We can have our vision of healing, build toward it with healing treatments, but the results will come in their own time. God, as healing energy, appears when the unconscious mind is prepared to receive it. *"If you build it, He will come."* Persistence and patience are required on our part. Results are to be left to God.

Part II

INSTRUCTIONS FOR HEALING

NOTE TO THE READER

The words "suggestive magnetic therapy or treatments," "magnetic healing," and "suggestive therapeutics" as used herein are synonymous.

This pertains also to the words "suggestion" and "affirmation." Suggestion and affirmation in the context of this book mean the verbal suggestions given to the person receiving healing treatments when he or she is in the relaxed, receptive state.

Throughout the text I have used the word "subject" instead of "patient" or "client" to refer to the person receiving the healing treatment. I have done so because it is more appropriate in treatments among family and friends. Only in the addendum are the words patient and client used.

4

PREPARATION FOR HEALING

Preparation is vital to creating conditions in which healing can happen. Discussed here are a number of ways which can help prepare you to do healing treatments. Allow a little time each day for praying, meditating, thinking about God, and directing those activities toward the treatment. Ideally, one should begin preparation a day or two before the treatment. A few minutes of meditation to center oneself just prior to a treatment session is also important and will be discussed again later.

Any normal, healthy person will be able to do suggestive magnetic therapy provided he or she understands the philosophy in Part 1 and prepares for giving treatments as discussed in this section. With understanding, preparation, and practice one can become competent at creating a healing environment.

Preparation should be a pleasure. Prayer, meditation, reading the Bible, and contemplating God are enjoyable and inspiring experiences. What may be difficult is finding time for these things in a busy daily schedule or routine, especially because it involves periods of uninterrupted concentration. It is, however, well worth the effort to make preparation for healing a priority. For how prepared you are may well determine the success of the healing treatments you give.

Our approach to suggestive magnetic therapy is a spiritual one. We will keep the experience in a spiritual context for reasons already cited. Therefore, the preparation exercises and recommendations included here are spiritual disciplines which you may already practice. However, we will use these disciplines specifically as preparation for healing sessions.

While both healer and subject should prepare to create the best environment for healing, the major responsibility falls on the facilitator. Treatments usually take 20 to 30 minutes. During that time the healing facilitator is responsible for sustaining a healing atmosphere. He or she is active and focused throughout the treatment session while the subject need only be in a relaxed receptive state.

Preparation serves the same purpose for musicians, athletes, public speakers, and anyone who requires preparation to give one's best. However, unlike activities such as sports and music, preparation for healing involves spiritual grounding. So our preparation involves mostly consciousness-raising activities.

The healing environment can best be established when the healer's preparation efforts focus on the healing process and his subject and not on himself as facilitator. The more focused you are on God, the healing process, and the person receiving the treatment, the more successful the session will likely be. The better you are able to focus on those things, the less you will be conscious of self. That is to say the more immersed you can become in the healing process, the more your subject will benefit.

It is somewhat similar to public speaking. The better one knows the subject matter and makes it relevant to the audience's interest or needs, the more successful will be his or her talk. Of all the fears people have, public speaking ranks at the top of the list. Yet, if the speaker's focus is not on himself but on his topic and his audience, his speech will have much better chance of being successful—if success is defined not as how well a speaker is received, but how well his subject matter is received and the way it affects the audience. The success of the speaker thus depends on his interest in, and knowledge of, his topic and his empathy with the audience.

Suggestive magnetic therapy is, however, unlike public speaking in one respect. Public speaking can be a terrifying experience for those who are unprepared and whose attention is centered on themselves and not their subject. There have been cases where people have had heart attacks while giving speeches, so stressful is the situation. Few facing public speaking engagements do so with complacency. Even experienced speakers get "butterflies," but learn to use them to their advantage as a spur to make sure they prepare.

Such is not the case with healing treatments. For while preparation is necessary for healing with suggestive magnetic therapy, doing the treatments should not be a fearful situation. It should always be just the opposite. It is an experience both healer and the subject must look forward to. If they do not look forward to the treatment session, then something is amiss, and the treatment should be canceled or postponed. The healer must be prepared mentally and physically and have adequate physical energy, otherwise the treatment may do more harm than good. Both facilitator and subject must expect the session to be a positive, uplifting happening. Preparation helps to insure that this happens.

As the object of your healing treatments will most likely be a friend or relative, "stage fright" should not be a factor. However, suggestive magnetic therapy does create an uncommon relationship between the healer and subject. It is a unique experience because God is sustained as a center of attention throughout the healing session at a very personal level. In a sense it is practicing the presence of God so that healing can happen.

Entering this event, the facilitator may feel a bit awkward, especially when stating the affirmation. For it is not an ordinary verbal communication. When you, as facilitator, repeat a suggestion, you are not talking to the person's conscious mind, but to the subconscious and to God, the Creative Force within him. You may feel somewhat uncomfortable in doing so. This will no doubt be the closest you come to stage fright in the healing experience. But this nervousness should quickly pass as you turn your mind away from self to God. This is accomplished with proper and adequate preparation.

Preparation will clear out unwanted debris from the mind and replace it with a positive attitude, and spiritual support. It is preparation which will get our "little selves" out of the way. We permit God access as we remove the obstacles to healing.

Healing is a natural function of Creative Energy, of God, and naturally occurs to the degree that we are able to attune to God. *"Let that mind be in you, that was [is] in Christ."* (Phil. 2:5). That is, our mind is to be in harmony with God. God cannot be coerced into healing.

"...all healing comes of the Lord, and there is not anything you may do save attune the body forces...to the awareness that God is, and is creative in its very purpose." (3042-1)

By removing mental and emotional barriers—doubt, fear, resentment, selfishness—and replacing such attitudes with the "mind of Christ," we create a healing environment.

Contemplating God

Edgar Cayce also tells us that just considering God, as healing energy, as electrical vibration within us, raises the very energy we're thinking about to its creative healing level:

... The force in nature that is called electrical... is that same force ye worship as Creative or God in action!

Seeing this, feeling this, knowing this, ye will find that not only does the body become revivified, but by the creating in every atom of its being the knowledge of the activity of this creative force or principal as related to spirit, mind, body – all three are renewed. For these are as the Trinity in the body, these are as the Trinity in the principles of the very life force itself – as the Father, the Son, the Spirit—the Body, the Mind, the Spirit—these are one. One God, one activity. Then see him, know him, in those influences. For even as the Son gave, "I of myself may do nothing, but as the father working in me, through me." *So it is with an individual entity or soul that sees the activities which man has been given in the earth. For the first command is ever as thine own,* "Be ye wise and subdue the earth." (1299-1)

This awareness of God manifesting as electrical vibration is a revolutionary thought. It broadens our definition of God and throws light on the biblical statement that, *"the body is the temple of the living God."* (I Cor. 6:19)

Without God functioning in the body as electricity, we would not exist. Even cursory readings in physiology reveal electricity's pervasive activity in a physical body. For example, the heart receives continuous electrical stimulation which prompts its beating. If the heart does not receive the correct electrical stimulation, an artificial pacemaker can be installed to provide the required electrical impulses without which the heart would cease to function. Our bodies function because of the electrical activity within them. We are saturated with the electrical vibrations: *"... In him we live, and move, and have our being."* (Acts 17:28)

Our attunement is enhanced by considering that this life energy is within us as well as every living thing. Our preparation for healing is strengthened by this new perspective of God. Seeing this aspect of God does not lessen our respect or reverence for him. Just the opposite; it agrees with what the Bible says about the body being the temple of God and does so in a concrete way. This perspective goes beyond just believing that somewhere inside of us, the elusive spirit of God resides. He is life itself and permeates every atom, every cell of our bodies. Thus the belief that God as omnipresent takes on new meaning.

When you contemplate God, consider this omnipresence. Focus also on God's healing qualities. Think about the electrical vibrations in the atoms and cells of every living thing. Realize that your thoughts, prayers, affirmations, and hands emit or create vibrations. And that these very same vibrations can affect the vibrations of the atoms in the person you are treating. Consider these and other relevant ideas as a preparation discipline. You will later find that this is also the frame of mind you will want to be in when you are doing suggestive magnetic treatments. For these vibrations to be such that they help create a healing environment, God, as well as your healing intention, must be focused upon throughout the treatments you give.

Concentration

Ability to concentrate is required in suggestive magnetic therapy. When doing treatments you must be able to concentrate on the healing intention and God, to the exclusion of irrelevant and negative thoughts. Meditation seeks to eliminate all thought while focusing on a word, affirmation, sound, or the breath. Concentration, unlike meditation, invites, thoughts relevant to the subject being concentrated upon.

For example, a student trying to solve a particular test problem would try to keep his attention on the subject at hand. Thoughts not pertinent the problem are pushed aside, leaving the mind free to consider the problem, the question.

Try this simple exercise in concentration; pick up a nearby object, a pencil, for instance. Think about its shape, size, color, and what it is made from, where its raw materials came from, and what processes the materials went through to finally become a pencil. This is a simple enough task and easy to do.

Not quite so simple or easy is the task of concentrating on a particular line of thinking. In doing healing treatments you must concentrate not on tangible things, but on words, images, or spiritual concepts relevant to healing. All thoughts the healer entertains must be relevant to, and originate from, his healing intention. When other thoughts appear, he must eliminate them by replacing them with healing thoughts.

Try this exercise: use one of your house plants to practice on. If there is a part of the plant that is wilted or a leaf or other part damaged, make it your intention to help that heal. If the plant is healthy in all respects, make it your intention to help the plant continue to grow and prosper. Your intention is simply the purpose of your thoughts and actions. Think to yourself: "My purpose is to create an environment in which healing can occur in this plant." Consider the life force in the plant, its electrical nature, and its electrical vibrations. Bear in mind that your positive thoughts, attitudes, and emotions contribute to the healing environment. They affect the vibrations of the plant as they are directed to it. Touch the plant.

As you think about the electrical life force—God—in the plant, as you concentrate on this and other healing thoughts, bring your attention to your hand touching the plant while maintaining your line of thinking. Feel the energy in your hand. Energy flows to where your attention is focused. Your thoughts flow as vibrations, through your hand to the plant. Your whole body vibrates to the thoughts you think. Thought produces vibration which affects living things around you as you direct your thoughts to them and when you touch them. Continue to touch the plant, all the while retaining your healing intention and thoughts. The source of life in the plant is the electrical influence in its atoms. It is the same source of life and all things including you. Both your plant and you are filled with the same life force manifesting as electrical vibration at the atomic level. Thus you and your plant have the same basic building blocks of life. Consider this oneness, this thing you have in common with your plant. Then consider how your positive thoughts—your intention—allows that God force to do its natural function of healing.

Bible reading

Read the Four Gospels which tell of the life of Jesus. They speak not only to our conscious mind, but also to our unconscious. There is much here that is applicable to daily living. The precepts that Jesus taught are sound psychological advice for healthy mental attitudes. Then, too, there is much beauty and mysticism which speaks to our inner selves in the Gospels, especially in St. John.

Reading John, chapters fourteen to seventeen, is recommended by Edgar Cayce. Some of what is said in these chapters is easily understood, while other parts may not be consciously understood. Nonetheless, it nourishes both one's conscious mind and   inner mind and spirit.

By reading the Four Gospels, our fate in healing is also strengthened. Many healings are described therein. As you read these, you will notice that Jesus used his healing hands and healing words—techniques that we employ in suggestive magnetic therapy.

Whether or not you are more inclined to read with a critical eye for what is readily understood, or if you read primarily for its inspirational value, the Bible will aid in your preparation for healing by strengthening your faith.

No matter how often the Gospels are read, they seem to remain fresh, to be living words. And often what we read becomes better understood by re-reading. Sometimes it speaks to us more clearly at one time than another because it addresses a problem or experience we are having in our lives.

Bible reading, especially the New Testament, should be a regular part of your preparation for healing. It will influence your prayers, meditation, and contemplation and enhance your attunement for healing.

Prayer

Pray without ceasing. This is what you do during the suggestive magnetic treatments. For the healing environment requires that the healer sustains communication with the Divine within the person who is the object of the treatment.

Prayer is talking to God. The healer communicates with his intention, laying on of hands, and verbal suggestions or affirmations. He also needs to talk to God as preparation for healing, just prior to the healing sessions

One way is, of course, to use traditional prayers, such as the Lord's Prayer (Matt. 6:9-13; Luke 11:1-4), and the Twenty-Third Psalm. The latter is a form of affirmation, which acknowledges the ways we rely on God for strength and guidance. The Lord's Prayer is supplication to God, to act in one's life. These two prayers are different, but complement each other.

Use prayer in your preparation for healing to express your needs and concerns regarding the treatments you are to give. Think about the particular treatment and person you seek to aid. Blanket that healing experience in prayer beforehand. Surround the place of treatment with positive, protective prayer. One prayer for protection which Cayce gave goes something like this: *"As I open myself to those unseen forces that surround the throne of grace and beauty and might, I throw about myself the protection that comes with the thought of the Christ."* Prayers of protection serve to keep negative influences out of your own consciousness and out of the place used for healing.

Another simple prayer, which is part of a longer prayer attributed to St. Francis, is, *"Make me an instrument of Thy peace."* We might add, *"... And Thy healing."* This is a simple but powerful prayer. Several years ago I was in a spiritual study group in which there was some tension among the participants. As the tension mounted, the simple prayer came to my mind and I silently repeated it myself. As soon as I did so, a noticeable vibration started at the end of my spine and moved quickly upward. It had a very calming effect on me. I felt no other noticeable effect than the physical sensation the peaceful feeling accompanying it.

"When you pray, do not use the vain repetition," Christ advised. (Matt. 6:7). Be sincere, concerned about the physical welfare of your subject. Express this in your prayers. Pray that any doubts you may have about healing be resolved. Acknowledge to yourself and God that it is God that heals and that you can only make conditions favorable for healing to happen. Pray for God to help you create this healing environment.

Self doubt, fear, and all negative thoughts thwart the healing experience. Use prayer to resolve any negative influences before you go into the healing situation. Even if you cannot remove these hindrances permanently from your mind, you can at least temporarily remove them during the healing session. Do not do a treatment if you cannot rid yourself of doubts and fears, whether or not these have to do with the healing experience or some other activity in your life. You must gain confidence that if you cannot seem to eliminate negativity from the thinking, God can. If you continue to prepare properly with prayer, meditation, and application of spiritual truths in your life, then unhealthy attitudes will give way to fate and confidence.

One need not be a saint to do suggestive magnetic therapy. We have our Creator to thank that each of us is given the potential for healing. What is required of us to heal or be healed is to remove those things that obstruct healing. If water will not flow through a pipe because of obstructions, we need only remove the obstructions. The water will then be free to flow. Prayer can help remove negative influences that block God's healing energy.

Meditation

While prayer is talking to God, meditation is listening to God. This listening to God means to be still, quiet the mind, *"be still and know, that I am God."* (Ps. 46:10). The object of meditation is not to hear God speak to us in words. He speaks to us, rather, in a still, small voice, or a knowing, rather than hearing. Meditation puts the mind in a state which allows God to move closer to our conscious awareness. It is a temporary melting, if you will, of human consciousness and the Universal Mind or Consciousness.

The meditator should be content simply to attain a quietness, a stilling of mental activity, and not to expect any sensational experience to occur. A common result of meditation is a peacefulness of the conscious mind. This experience can carry over into one's daily life. One way to approach meditation is with the attitude of simply spending quiet time with God, with no demands or expectations.

There should be no distractions during meditation, which would disrupt your concentration. Choose a room where you will not be disturbed and where noises are at a minimum. Allow ten to fifteen minutes for a meditation period. Shorter times are okay. I t is not necessary to spend much longer times in meditation. Meditation is not used by the suggestive magnetic therapy facilitator during the treatment itself. The purpose of meditation is to attune to God; to remove our awareness from the outer world to our source of life within.

Two methods of meditation which are suited for our preparation purposes are meditation upon an affirmation, and meditation on a single word or sound. Both of these methods require that we first make our bodies physically comfortable. A simple way of doing this, which still allows meditation to work is to sit upright in a comfortable chair with the spine straight. This sitting position allows the creative energy within us to move up the spine to the higher spiritual centers in the body. Sitting in a slumped position tends to block the movement of this energy. Also, to allow the blood to circulate freely, it is helpful to loosen belts and shoelaces or to take off your shoes.

Try this exercise to get a feel for the posture and position you should be in for meditation. Rest your hands on your lap with palms up. Close your eyes and become aware of your body. If there is any physical tension, try to relax the area involved. Turn your attention to your breathing. Begin to take long, slow breaths. As you do this, feel the tension draining from your body. Become aware of the expansion and contraction of your abdomen as you breathe. Let your shoulders slump in relaxation, releasing any tension there. Continue to be aware of the peacefulness this long, slow breathing brings. You may notice that when your attention is on one part of your body the energy seems to increase there. Move your attention to your hands. You will likely notice the energy in your palms first. Be aware of that for a few moments. Then move your attention to the back of your hands. Continue to direct your attention to different areas of your body. Each time you redirect your awareness to a different area the energy will seem to increase there.

After a minute or two of relaxing your body in this way, you will be physically prepared to meditate.

A basic meditation method is to focus on a single word or sound. With your eyes closed focus on the word "one." Listen to the sound of the word. Concentrate on the word, the sound, to the exclusion of all other thoughts. When other thoughts do creep in, simply bring your attention back to the sound of "one."

There is no magic in the word itself. It is only an object to focus upon for stilling the mind. When the conscious mind is quiet, the universal mind can get through. *"Be still and know..."* Do not expect to hear God. Neither expect anything specific to happen at the conscious level during meditation. But know that meditation contributes to your preparation for healing and enriches your life. When used, just prior to the healing experience, it brings a peaceful, calming effect, both physically and mentally to the healing facilitator.

When the word, the sound, is followed, there will come a point where you momentarily lose yourself in silence. Then, suddenly, you will become aware again of thoughts and words. When this happens, we focus on the word-sound. You are closest to God in the stillness between the words. It is somewhat like the white space between printed words. For example: when in meditation you focus on slowly repeating, *"One, one, one, one, one-nnnn,"* you reach a point where there is silence; that space between the repeating of the word in your mind. This silence, the space, can stretch out as, "One, one, one............. one..." You do not force this space. It just occurs at times without your immediately realizing it. During this emptiness the conscious mind makes contact with the Universal Mind. It may also be a time *"when the subconscious [temporarily becomes], the conscious mind, and when the universal forces are made active in subconsciousness."* (900-31)

End your meditation by bringing your attention back to your body. Take a few deep breaths and begin moving your body to allow the blood to circulate normally again. Avoid jumping up quickly. Instead, take your time reorienting yourself. Stretching should help make you alert again.

The second meditation method you may wish to use as preparation for healing is one that focuses on an affirmation. Rather than listening to a single word or sound, meditation, with an affirmation requires repeating one or more sentences addressed to God. An example is, *"Create in me a pure heart, O God. Make me an instrument of Thy peace and healing."* Such, affirmations sound much like prayers. The difference is in how they are used. When used in meditation the words are focused on and repeated several times. The meanings of the words reflect the purpose of the meditation. After the affirmation is said internally or aloud, the meditator sits in the silence for several minutes—letting God "speak" within.

Try this meditation method using the following affirmation: *"The Lord is my shepherd, I shall not want."* But, first, follow the suggestions given earlier to physically prepare your body for meditation. When your body is relaxed and ready, begin to concentrate on the affirmation. Repeat it to yourself slowly, letting the words sink into your unconscious. Take your time. Leave a few seconds between each repeating of the affirmation. Say the affirmation at least three times or a few more times if you feel moved to do so. Then silence your thoughts. Let your mind rest.

At this point focus your attention to the area inside your forehead. Do not concentrate on any particular physical part. Remain mentally silent. This is the time the Universal Forces become active just below your conscious level. The better you are able to block out distractions and thoughts, the more you will be centered. Should you become distracted, bring your awareness back to the space inside your forehead. If distractions continue in the form of thoughts, repeat the affirmation to regain your focus.

After you have been able to maintain the silence for several minutes, you may wish to direct prayers to those about whom you are concerned. Prayers for healing at this time are recommended. Direct your prayer as you normally would. Or you may visualize the person surrounded by white light. As you do this, have your hands resting on your lap, palms up, but not touching each other. This is a way of directing the spiritual energy raised to those for whom you pray. During meditation, however, you may wish to have your hands in your lap, palms up, with your right hand resting on your left (vice versa if left-handed.)

End this meditation, the same way you did with the first meditation method by bringing your attention back to your body. Take your time getting up, then do some stretching and moving about to restore your blood circulation to normal. Feelings of restfulness, peace, and well-being are normal aftereffects of meditation. During meditation your breath can become almost imperceptible. Such is the calming effect of meditation. When you come out of meditation, be sure you are fully awake and your body alert, especially if you plan to drive or do anything that requires your full attention.

If you are inexperienced at meditation, the first method discussed—using one word-sound—will probably be easiest to do. Though quite simple it is nonetheless very fruitful. Not just beginners but also the most advanced meditators often use this method.

Visualization

This is the only part of the preparation that is more useful to the person seeking healing than for the healing facilitator. For, while the healer may use it for "rehearsing" the treatment sessions, the subject for healing can use it to help him accept the possibility of being healed.

As facilitator it is helpful to visualize yourself doing a treatment for a particular person's ailment. If you do many treatments with the same person over a number of days, it may only be necessary to visualize the first few treatments. After that the procedure and the worded suggestions should be well familiar to you and visualization would be unnecessary. However, for every treatment you should still always prepare with prayer and meditation. And you may visualize, or picture, the person and place of the treatment when you pray and meditate, especially when you pray a prayer of protection or envision a white light around the healing situation.

To familiarize yourself with a particular healing treatment you may rehearse it visually. Picture the person and place of the treatment. Visualize yourself going through each step of the treatment process. First, see yourself relaxing your subject with a simple back and shoulder massage and/or words intended to relax him mentally and physically. Next, picture yourself with hands resting on the person's back and head. Then imagine yourself repeating the suggestion, word for word. As you visualize the treatment keep in mind that your role in the healing process is to create a healing environment. You are not expected to know these procedures well enough to do them yet. They are mentioned here because of the visualization that should be a part of your preparation for healing. The steps and procedures used in suggestive magnetic therapy are explained in detail in the next three chapters. Then in Chapter 8 we will talk you through a complete healing treatment.

Visualization serves a different purpose for the person who is to receive the healing treatments. She can help the facilitator by coming to each session mentally prepared. By using visualization she can condition her mind, both consciously and unconsciously, to be receptive to healing. As facilitator, you should instruct your subject in the visualization technique and encourage her to practice it. The more the subject believes that she can be healed, the more she contributes to the healing environment. And it makes a healing facilitator's role easier. If, on the other hand, the subject comes for a treatment clouded with doubt and fear, or negativity, your chances of helping her are slim.

It is true that the purpose of suggestion, and of getting yourself into a relaxed state, is to bypass the conscious mind's inharmonious attitudes and get into the sub-conscious mind. Nonetheless, your subject can aid this process by doing as much as she can to contribute to the healing process. Visualization can be a major tool for implementing belief within the subject.

How does visualization work, and how can the subject of your treatments use it? To understand how it works, we must consider how it affects the subconscious mind. In the chapter, "The Subconscious and Healing," we noted how visualization improved accuracy of basketball shooters. By mentally picturing themselves scoring baskets—without even touching a basketball—they improved their skills. How is this possible? The subconscious cannot tell the difference between what is real and what is vividly imagined. The subconscious seems to accept messages of actual happenings via our five senses and imagined visual scenes flavored with the appropriate emotions. What the subconscious receives it accepts. It has no reasoning powers. This is why visualization can be a great aid in healing. Because the unconscious mind controls the functioning of the body, visualization can influence the subconscious and therefore implement or enhance the healing process.

To be most effective visualization must see the desired result rather than the process of getting to the goal. Unlike taking a scenic drive to a country place where "half the fun is getting there," or enjoying the drive, visualization works best when the "getting there" is left out. Focus instead on being there now. See your destination, your goal, having already been reached. Leave it to the subconscious to make it possible, remembering that when the subconscious can accept healing, it opens itself and the body to the higher vibrations of the Creator.

Let's say, for example, that the subject of your healing treatments seeks to cure arthritis. Rather than visualizing herself getting treatments from you and her doctor, or taking drugs, she instead should see herself using the affected parts as if they were healthy and normal. If the arthritis is in her hands, she could see herself doing things with them that she did before the onset of arthritis, or see herself doing things that she would like to be able to do in the future. She might also picture her doctor telling her in amazement that he finds no trace of her problem remaining. That somehow it has healed by itself.

The visualization technique should become a regular part of your subject's preparation for healing. The severity of the problem and how sincere the subject's desire is to overcome it could determine how frequently visualization might be done. A logical and practical time to do it would be at the same time one does prayer and meditation.

The Bible advises us, *"... without vision the people perish* (Prov. 29:18). We can improvise and say, "With visualization we prosper." To the subconscious seeing is believing. Help those you give treatments to understand this and encourage them to use visualization.

Forgiveness

Forgiveness helps healing happen. *"Forgive us our debts as we forgive our debtors."* (Matt. 6:12) Debts, not in the financial sense, but resentments, grudges, and hate congeal in our own physical makeup. Hate directed toward us from another person does not affect us nearly as seriously as does our own hate for another. Our conscious attitudes affect our physical condition. Cayce said that we cannot hate our neighbor without having stomach problems. Forgiveness may well resolve the same physical problems that hate causes.

Before coming into a healing treatment, both healer and subject would do well to become aware of any negative attitudes he or she may harbor toward others. Of course, suggestive magnetic therapy should never be done if there are ill feelings between healer and subject. Such attitudes must be resolved before a treatment, otherwise it will do more harm than good. It is the responsibility of both healer and subject to do their own mental/spiritual housecleaning. They must both come to the treatment session with "good vibes," so to speak.

How does one forgive? Obviously, prayer is the most practical way. While going to the person one needs to forgive may sometimes be best, such is not always the case, nor is it always practical. Sometimes forgiving persons who you feel wronged you may fall on deaf ears.

They may not be receptive or may not even realize they had done anything that warranted your forgiveness. In such cases, the problem exists only in your own mind and can be dealt with through prayer. If a person hates you without good reason, the problem is in that person's mind. And you should avoid falling into the trap of hating or condemning that one in return. Rather, do what you can with prayer and goodwill, then release a situation to God.

It is another situation altogether if you find yourself hating. Then you must renew your mind spiritually. You must take action to resolve the attitude before seeking to facilitate healing or to be the subject of healing treatments.

Hate, resentments, and ill will constrict one's consciousness, limit freedom of expression, and inhibit wellness of the physical body. It is practically impossible to attribute a particular ailment to a specific attitude or action. And that may be a good thing. For if we knew that an attitude we had toward an individual caused us a particular physical problem we might try to resolve our attitude toward that person only, when we should, instead, deal with that attitude as it relates to all people.

We would do well to forgive ourselves also as preparation for healing. Unless we do so, we may feel guilty and unworthy of healing. We must never feel that way. We should take responsibility for own conscious attitudes and try our best to overcome negative ones. But guilt serves no useful purpose. All deserve healing. We are not expected to be saints. You can search the New Testament from one end to the other, but not find one instance where Jesus turned anyone away who sought healing from Him. His attitude was, *"...neither do I judge thee."* (John 8:11)

In truth, we judge and treat ourselves as we treat and judge others. It may not appear to be the case, but it is a spiritual truth. Christ could have said, "You do unto yourself as you do unto others," because the golden rule not only influences our soul's destiny but also our life here and now.

Pray to forgive others and yourself. Pray the Lord's Prayer. Visualize white light around those you need to forgive, or do whatever works for you in putting aside negative thoughts. Do this until you know the situations are resolved in your consciousness. If they are not completely resolved, you must at least be able to set them aside temporarily and come to the treatment with an attitude of goodwill and a positive healing consciousness. This is the purpose of preparation.

5

THE HEALING ENVIRONMENT

—

Several things must be considered before getting into the treatment itself. First is preparation, which was covered in the last chapter. Then there is the place, the room and which the treatment will be done. And, just prior to treatment, the subject must be put into a relaxed, passive state which will allow his or her unconscious mind to respond to suggestion and magnetic healing. The next two chapters explain in detail suggestion and magnetic healing, the heart of suggestive magnetic therapy and the healing environment. This chapter deals with preparing the physical and mental environment up to the point that suggestion and laying on of hands are done.

The physical location

Since your subject will have his or her eyes closed during the session, the visual appearance of the room is of little importance. However, sounds and smells can contribute to or distract from the treatment.

Smells are not usually a problem. However, if there are offensive smells in the room, you may wish to use an air freshener. Any fragrance that is agreeable to both healer and subject could be used. If you do choose to use an air freshener, use only enough to cover the offensive smell. Even a pleasant aroma, if too strong, may detract from the healing process. I prefer not to use incense for this reason. A rule of thumb might be to never use any air freshener unless offensive odors are present in the treatment room.

If conditions are right treatments can be done outdoors, weather and temperature permitting. However, indoors there is much less chance of unexpected disturbances such as curious visitors, insects, or noises.

Unwanted sounds can disrupt concentration of the healing facilitator and possibly startle the subject out of his relaxed state. Doors and windows should be shut to minimize sounds from outside the treatment room. Relaxing music may be played which could enhance the healing environment and help to mute outside sounds. Choose soothing music or recorded nature sounds with no vocals and play the music at a low volume to enhance relaxation. Cayce said that waltzes were music favorable for healing. Of course, the music chosen should be agreeable to both healer and subject. Use music only to enhance the physical environment and help the subject stay relaxed. Consider using the same music when you do repeated sessions for the same person over a period of time. In so doing, your subject will begin to associate a particular piece of music with healing. His mind, then, should more rapidly move into the relaxed, passive state.

Physical equipment

A chair, stool, or padded table, such as a massage table will be needed for the person receiving treatment. Sidney Weltmer recommended use of a stool or a padded table. Which works best will depend largely on the physical condition of your subject and his ailment. If he finds it comfortable to sit on a stool, that would be best in most situations. The reason is, first, that in this position the spine is easiest to reach, and second, the facilitator will find it more convenient to walk around the sitting subject than to walk around a table with him lying on it. In most treatments you will have one hand on your subject's spine at least part of the time. Chairs that are high backed make this virtually impossible.

There is one possible disadvantage when the subject sits on a stool. Without support, the back may get cramped from being in one position throughout the treatment. A stool with a lower back support would solve this for most people. However, for many people this is not a problem. I have had people doze off during treatment while they sat on a stool that had no back support. When choosing to have your subject sit or recline keep in mind that you may need to place one hand on the spine at least some of the time during a healing session.

Treatments often require that the healing facilitator remain in one position for five minutes or more. During this time a stool is practical for him to use. He can alternate standing and sitting to avoid being cramped or tired. The person receiving the treatment has the option of dozing off, but the facilitator must remain alert, focused, and active.

Agreement

You have, no doubt, heard the phase, "I ate something that didn't agree with me." When you eat something that doesn't agree with you, it does often make you sick. Naturally, when you do something that is not healthy— that your body finds disagreeable—it reacts. For instance, excessive exposure to the sun is disagreeable to the skin and can cause sunburn and skin cancer.

Psychosomatic illness is a term used for real or imagined physical problems caused by attitude and emotions. "It's all in your head," we are told; meaning that the body is disagreeing with thoughts to the extent that they detrimentally affect the body's health. The prescribed cure is to stop the disagreeable thoughts and replace them with agreeable ones. It's another way of saying our thinking is producing vibrations that are either in or out of harmony with life-enhancing forces in the physical body.

In suggestive magnetic therapy, agreement is the two minds holding the same healing purpose. That is, the intention in the mind of the healer verbalized in the form of suggestion and transferred to the mind and body of the subject. This constitutes agreement. Agreement of this healing thought in the two minds is essential to the healing environment.

Agreement cannot be over emphasized. Sidney Weltmer's healing philosophy was based on agreement as were the methods he used. He was inspired by Matthew 18:19, *"... if two of you shall agree on earth as touching anything that they shall ask, it shall be done for them of my Father which is in heaven."* Weltmer interpreted this to mean that when the minds of two or more people are in harmony and agreement, then creative vibrations are raised and healing can happen. Weltmer structured his healing techniques to implement his healing philosophy. In suggestive magnetic therapy, we endeavor to have the unconscious mind of the subject accept the suggestion or affirmation from the healer. Two minds are then in agreement, both having the same intention or purpose at the same time.

Agreement should also be the guiding attitude of the healer toward the subject of his or her treatments. Before the treatment, and as a treatment is being done, the facilitator should communicate with the subject in a totally positive way. He should refrain from using any negative words. For example, instead of saying, *"Don't open your eyes during the treatment,"* he should rephrase the statement into a positive one: *"With your eyes closed throughout the treatment, you'll be more relaxed and receptive to healing."* While this may seem trivial, it really is not. Your attitude toward your subject must be cooperative, rather than domineering. The facilitator should never act or talk in a superior manner to the person with whom he is working. He must not have the attitude that, *"You are the ailing person and I am the healer."* For in truth, the facilitator's job is only to make conditions possible which allow God to find expression in healing. With reverence and respect for Creative Forces, the facilitator sees himself simply as assuming the temporary role of healing facilitator. You, as facilitator, will soon discover that it is a privilege to take on this role, for your subject is allowing you to assume the role, this opportunity, which is mutually rewarding for both of you.

Any bossy, negative, or otherwise disagreeable words or attitudes can create tension between participants and prohibit the healing environment from being established. In one Cayce reading he was asked if a mother could do the healing treatments for her child. His answer was "no" because of some unresolved conflict between the two. Unless such friction is resolved, more harm than good would result from treatments.

Just remembering that suggestive magnetic therapy is a spiritual experience helps participants cooperate. The facilitator sets the atmosphere or tone of the experience from start to finish. If he or she has prepared for the treatment with prayer, meditation, as advised in the last chapter, then the treatment will reflect this preparation.

Intention

Three main elements constitute Weltmer's healing method: intention, suggestion, and laying on of hands. The latter two, as mentioned previously, are the subjects of the next two chapters.

Intention is reflected in the verbal suggestion as well as being conveyed through the hands. And intention is the thoughts focused upon throughout a treatment session. Treatment begins with the facilitator holding in his mind the intention to relax the subject. After his subject has become relaxed enough to start the magnetic healing and suggestions, then the facilitator changes his intention to a healing theme rather than a relaxing one.

It would seem obvious that we should know our intention is to create a healing environment. However, it is emphasized here because it must be concentrated on throughout the entire session. Concentration was discussed in the last chapter, but because of its importance in maintaining the intention we bring it up again. Without the ability to concentrate one cannot become an effective facilitator. Any wavering from the specific healing purpose breaks the mental connection of the healing thought from facilitator to subject. If concentration on the attention is broken, the healing environment is weakened or lost. It is a matter of training the mind to concentrate on one central theme.

In our fast-paced technological world we are seldom focused for long periods of time. We have become impatient TV channel-and Internet-surfers. Yet, we have within us the need and ability to center ourselves, to become less scattered. Meditation has become a great asset to us in this respect, and an oasis for our mind and spirit.

Concentrating on our healing intention is somewhat like focusing on an affirmation for meditation. The main difference is that the healing intention is directed to the subject rather than being held within.

During a typical suggestive magnetic therapy session, the facilitator repeats the suggestion three to six times. At this time focusing on the intention is easiest because it is spoken. The time between the repeating of the suggestion is when we rely most on our powers of concentration, because it is then that extraneous thoughts can slip into our conscious minds distracting us from our intention. Even if the distracting thoughts are not negative ones, they nonetheless dilute the healing intention. For example, I had a workshop participant ask if she should tell her subject the psychic impressions she felt she was getting regarding her subject. While these may be fascinating, they have no place in the treatment, no matter how good they may seem. If the facilitator's mind is occupied on sending the healing intention to her subject's subconscious, there should be no interference from irrelevant thoughts.

Should interfering thoughts become a problem, remind yourself of the purpose of the treatment, and focus on the healing intention. One way to do this is to have the intention written out and placed where you can see it while you do treatments. If necessary you can repeat or read it to yourself. Sometimes I print the words of the suggestion in large letters and put it where I can easily see it. Then it is visible to me when I want to repeat the suggestion and available for refocusing upon should irrelevant thoughts arise.

Centering the Facilitator

Just prior to beginning a treatment find a place where you can meditate and pray for few minutes. Use the meditation to "center" yourself, to become peaceful within yourself, and to reflect on the purpose of the treatment.

Remember your role remains the same regardless of the problem your subject is experiencing. Therefore, during this short meditation and prayer time, free yourself of earthly cares and reflect on your relationship with God. Remind yourself that God manifest as healing energy— electrical vibrations—and that you, as healing facilitator, seek to make the environment favorable for healing to happen. God already saturates our bodies electrically. We as facilitators seek to remove the obstructions which inhibit or prevent positive electrical vibrations from reaching the subconscious mind of our subject. Centering will help us accomplish this goal.

Relaxing Your Subject Verbally

As healing facilitator, you must help your subject into this relaxed, passive state physically and mentally. In his book, *The Relaxation Response*, Dr. Herbert Benson states, *"The passive attitude is perhaps the most important element in eliciting the relaxation response,"* or the positive, physical reaction to meditation. Sidney Weltmer felt that the mental state of these patients was of such importance that he devoted up to half of the treatment time for getting them into the passive, receptive state. When giving a half-hour treatment, he would spend half that time relaxing the patient, if it was required.

Do not make the beginner's mistake I did some years ago I when I told a subject to just go ahead and carry on a normal conversation with a friend as a treatment was being done. I didn't realize then that his subconscious would not be open and receptive to my healing efforts while his conscious mind was active.

Weltmer stated that the success of treatments depended on the belief and passivity of the subject, and the ability of the healing facilitator to concentrate on his healing intention.

Your subject may attain this passive state in several ways. Here are six methods you may choose from:

Method # 1: Bible reading to your subject

Method # 2: Dozing; your subject drifting into sleep (especially recommended by Cayce in the treatment of children)

Method # 3: Meditation done by the subject

Method # 4: Verbally relaxing the subject

Method #   5: Verbally relaxing the subject and having him tense and relax his muscles in the process

Method # 6: Massage of the subject's back and head

Method # 1

If your subject is a very religious person, she may be more receptive to Bible reading than the other methods of relaxation noted here. However, you may encourage her to relax physically and let the inspirational reading bring about peace of mind.

Choose verses from the New Testament which describe healings or that refer to the healing power of God. Read for fifteen minutes or so before beginning to do the laying on of hands magnetic treatment and suggestions. In at least one reading Cayce recommended reading the Bible as the treatment is being done. When this is done, the Bible reading would also serve as the suggestion. You may wish to try this. To do so, you will need to position your Bible where you can see and read it while you're given the treatment.

Method # 2

Cayce recommended suggestion and magnetic healing treatment for children as they drift to sleep. This is the simplest of all relaxing methods and requires little or no effort on the part of the healing facilitator, the parent. She would simply let her child doze off at bedtime as usual before beginning a treatment.

Method # 3

This method may be used for persons adept at doing a relaxing form of meditation. Your subject can use meditation in lieu of the other relaxation methods if he believes he can attain a passive, receptive state of consciousness. Of course, this is the purpose of meditation—to listen, to be receptive to God. *"Be still and know..."*

Meditation, correctly done then, would still the active, reasoning mind of your subject so that your treatment can access his subconscious mind. Give your subject about ten minutes to meditate before starting a suggestive magnetic treatment. Then approach him in a very quite manner so as not to disrupt his meditation. Gently place your hands on his upper back and shoulders to begin the treatment. He should remain in a meditative state during the treatment.

Method # 4

This is a relaxation technique using your voice to help your subject relax. It is given here as an example only. You should use your own words when talking the subject of your treatments into the relaxed state. Read the following aloud slowly to get a better feel for how it would sound when repeated to the person receiving a treatment. Y ou could also tape it as you read and play it back to hear how it sounds to you. Then rephrase it more to your liking for your own use. This is about a ten minute tape. Begin recording now:

"As I rest my hands on your back, begin to take deep, slow breaths—very long, deep breaths. Inhale the air all the way down to your stomach and feel it expand. Slowly exhale until all the air is completely out of your lungs. Listen to your breath as it leaves your nostrils, and then hold your breath for a moment or two before inhaling again.

"Now breathe in again slowly—a very long, deep breath, expanding your chest and abdomen as you inhale. Then, when you've inhaled as much air as you can, hold it for a moment before releasing it back up and out your nose.

"As I talk, just continue this slow, deep breathing, and at the end of each inhale and exhale, hold your breath just for a few seconds before continuing.

"As you continue breathing, bring your awareness to your face, your scalp, the back of your head, and neck. Be conscious of the energies there. Become aware of any tensions and relax the muscles there. Relax the muscles around and behind your eyes. Now relax the rest of your face including your jaw. Unclench your teeth so they are not touching. Relax your chin and neck. All tension drains down from your face and neck and scalp. Feel it draining down over your shoulders, down your arms, into your hands, and out your fingertips. Feel the energy in your fingers as the tension drains out. Your face, scalp, and neck, are completely relaxed and peaceful, very peaceful now.

"Bring your attention to your shoulders and let them droop, releasing any tension there. Be aware of your upper arms, your biceps, feel them relaxing, the tension draining down. Now you feel your elbows and lower arms relaxing as the tension drains through your arms and out of your fingertips. Your shoulders, your arms, elbows, and hands are relaxed as all tension has strained out through your fingertips. Your head, your face, your neck, shoulders, arms, hands, and fingertips, are all relaxed now.

"Feel the energy in your hands. There is also a sense of energy in your head, neck, shoulders, and arms, though they are completely relaxed. The more you relax the more you can feel this peaceful life energy. Bring your attention to your chest, your abdomen, your upper and lower back, and hips. Release all tension there, beginning with your chest. Feel the muscles there relax as you breathe deeply. All the muscles along your spine from the shoulders all away down your back are relaxing now. Feel them letting go of all the tightness and becoming peaceful and relaxed. Now your abdomen relaxes as you draw in long, deep breaths. Feel the energy in your back, your chest, and abdomen as the tension all drains out, down your legs and out your feet. You can feel the energy in your toes as the tension leaves your body.

"Become aware, now, of the peacefulness throughout your head, neck, shoulders, arms, and hands, and your chest, back, and abdomen. All the muscles there are relaxed, yet alive with the life-force that is God.

"Bring your attention now to your hips, buttocks, and your thighs. Feel all the tension drain out of them, down your legs and out the bottoms of your feet. You can feel this tension being drawn out of your buttocks, hips, and thighs. Feel it leaving the bottoms of your feet and out the tips of your toes.

"Now relax your knees, your lower legs, and ankles. All tension is draining out, being drawn out as the muscles relax. Feel all the energy now in your feet as a tension drains through them out the bottoms of your feet and toes. As this last bit of tension is being drawn out through your feet, they too become relaxed and peaceful, yet alive with life energy.

"Continue to draw in long, deep breaths slowly, peacefully. You are completely relaxed now from the top of your head to the tips of your fingers and toes. Feel that total peace throughout your body.

"As your body remains in this calmness, you can focus your mind now on a peaceful scene—a favorite nature scene. Choose a place in nature that is quiet and where you can enjoy being alone, and you can be at peace. Observe the lushness of the trees and grass. Notice the sounds of birds, the smells, and the fresh air. Breathe in the clean, cool, pure air. Continue to focus on this refreshing scene as the treatment begins. You find you can stay focused on this place throughout the treatment. Even as I repeat the affirmation you can remain in peaceful relaxation in this place of healing."

Method # 5

The following method is similar to the above method except that it requires your subject to tense then relax his muscles in order to bring himself into the relaxed state. This may be used for people who are usually very aggressive or assertive and find it difficult to relax. It will help them to participate in at least the initial part of the treatment process.

This is about a fifteen minute relaxation "script."

"Take several long, slow, deep breaths. Inhale slowly, deeply. Feel your chest expanding. Take this breath all the way down into your abdomen. Feel it expanding as you breathe in deeply, slowly, peacefully. Now, exhale very slowly, releasing the air at a slow pace. When all the air is exhaled, hold your breath for a few moments and feel of your body beginning to relax. Breathe again, inhaling deeply, slowly, peacefully. A long deep breath. Feel it expanding your chest, your lungs, your abdomen. Then, when you have a full breath, hold it a few moments as I count to three – one...two...three. Exhale very slowly through our nose. You can hear the sound of air through your nostrils as you exhale slowly. As you exhale, tighten your abdomen, forcing the air up and out through your nose. Now, when all the air is exhaled, hold your breath; hold it, hold it, hold it. Now breathe in slowly.

"Take deep breaths at your own natural pace. Let your breathing supply adequate oxygen to your body. Breathe in as deeply as necessary, and as slowly as you can. Slowly and deeply. Now continue this slow deep breathing. Inhale very, very slowly, feeling your breath reaching all away down into your abdomen, expanding your abdomen. You can feel tingling in your hands, and in your legs and feet as this breath is expanding deeper and deeper into your being.

"Now, as you exhale, feel your attention drawn back to your face, to your nostrils, where you can hear your breath exhaling. Continue this back and forth, inhaling and exhaling. Slowly inhale, feeling the energy in your hands, feet, legs, your lower arms, and shoulders. Each deep breath that you take is more relaxing to you. Now, as you began to exhale, bring your attention back to your face.

"Tense up your face, scrunch it up tightly. Tense the muscles in your face, your scalp, and in the back of your head and neck. Tense it all up—tight, tighter. Hold it, hold it. Now release it. Release all the tension—all the tension from your head, from your scalp, from your neck, from your face. All the tension drains out, down your body. Down your body it drains, out your fingertips and out your toes. Your face, head, and neck are now relaxed and serene, relaxed and serene.

"Now, tighten your shoulders, your chest, your biceps—tighten, tighten. Hold it, hold it, hold it. Now relax slowly, slowly relax your muscles. Relax very peacefully. Breathe deeply again. Exhale, and catch your breath. Your head, your face, and your scalp, your neck and your shoulders, your biceps are now all peacefully relaxed. All the tension has trained down your body and out your fingertips and toes.

"Now, this time, tighten your lower arms, and tighten your hands into fists. Tighten, tighten, and hold it. Hold this tension in your fist and lower arms. Hold it, hold it, hold it. Now release. Let your hands unfold, let your fingers uncurl. Feel the peace now that the tension is gone, all drained out. Feel the tingling in your hands as the tension has dissipated into thin air.

"Breathe deeply. Feel the energy in your hands, and down your lower body, in your knees and in your lower legs and feet. All the tension has trained out the bottoms of your feet into the floor and the earth below.

"Place your hands in your lap now, one hand on top of the other with palms up. Just let your hands relax there. Now, tighten your lower body, your hips, your buttocks, your thighs. Tighten, tense them up, tense them up—hold it, hold it. Now relax. Feel all that tension drain out. Let all that tension dissipate into thin air. Now, your body from your head to your knees is relaxed and peaceful.

"Breathe deeply again now to refresh your body from head to knees. Slowly, deeply, breathe in. Feel your shoulders droop and the energy tingling in your hands.

"Now, tense your feet. Curl your toes under. Tighten your feet and your lower legs up to your knees. You will find that as you do this your hips, your buttocks, thighs, may tense also. Just hold that tension for a moment. Hold it, hold it, hold it. Now relax. Let out a sigh of released tension, uncurl your toes, put your feet flat on the floor again, release all the tension in your lower body and legs and feet. Feel the tension draining out, out the bottoms of your feet into the earth.

"Your whole body is now relaxed so that you can feel the life forces flowing. Feel this energy, this relaxing, flowing, peaceful energy of life from your head to your toes. There is energy in the midst of this relaxation, this peace.

"Become aware of this energy throughout your body, while at the same time your body continues to be relaxed. Your shoulders droop as low as they naturally can. Your hands are peaceful now, yet tingling with this life force.

"Continue to breathe deeply throughout this whole treatment to re-energize your body and feel this life force within it.

"Bring your attention to your face now as you stay relaxed. And in your mind's eye, picture, if you will, a favorite place, a favorite scene from your past, a nature scene. It is a most beautiful and peaceful scene. The air is fresh, and you can smell the fragrances of flowers, freshness of clean air, the sounds of nature, of birds, of insects. And there is a warm, fresh breeze. You can see the trees and the grass gently swaying in the breeze. You can picture every detail now of this scene—the vegetation, a stream, the trees in the distance, and further out are peaceful, majestic mountains. You can feel the peaceful-ness of this healthy environment, invigorating, renewing your body.

"As you stay in this place, breathe in the fresh air, and con-tinue to hear nature's sounds. Now, as you gaze at the scene, you are deeply refreshed, renewed, and invigorated by the lushness of the countryside and beauty of the distant moun-tains.

"Feel the life energy in nature and in yourself as the music becomes a part of the scene, intensifying the details. Just relax and enjoy the scene. You can remain in this peaceful place throughout this treatment. Your mind is at peace, you are free of all cares, breathing in the fresh country air, listening to the peaceful sounds of nature.

"You can refocus on this scene anytime during this treatment. It is so real that you feel as though you are there. And as the treatment begins you can remain focused on this place. Let the energy of my hands intensify your awareness of this peaceful scene. And, when I speak the affirmation aloud, just remain focused on this nature scene. Let the affirmation sink deeply into your inner mind, into your subconsciousness, where healing happens, where God is."

Method # 6

If you are competent at doing massage, you can use it to get your subject into the passive state. You need not be a professional massage therapist to do this simple back, neck, and scalp massage. However, you should have at least some massage experience, otherwise the person you are working on may detect your inexperience and be unable to relax.

Do not use massage if your subject is bed ridden, ill, injured, or uncomfortable with the idea of being massaged. Choose, instead, to use one of the verbally relaxing techniques above.

This massage requires no removal of clothing, except that it could not be done through heavy clothes or a thick pullover. A shirt or blouse should pose no problem. Your subject should wear loose-fitting clothes so that blood circulation will not be hindered during the treatment. Have him loosen his belt and shoelaces. It would be a good idea also to have your subject remove metal jewelry, especially necklaces. If your subject is a woman, you will need to get her approval to do her scalp if she has a hairdo or has her hair in place with a comb. This massage can be done without including the scalp. However, scalp massage can be very relaxing for your subject and should be included if possible.

Before you begin, make sure your hands are clean and dry. Have your subject sit on a stool, the same as he would if you were relaxing him verbally rather than with massage. There should be no back to the stool, which would make lower back massage difficult.

Begin the massage by placing your hands on your subject's shoulders, letting them rest there for a few seconds, then start a kneading motion along the shoulders and across the shoulder blades. When massaging over and between the shoulder blades use your fingertips and the heel of your hand. Brace your subject's body with your left hand on his left shoulder and use your right hand to do the massage. (Vice versa if you are left-hande). Avoid massage on the edges of the shoulder blades. You may massage on and between the shoulder blades with fingertips and the heel of your hand.

Remember the purpose of this massage is to relax your subject. Keep this intention in mind during the massage. It will guide you as to the amount of pressure to use and what areas of the back to spend more time massaging.

After you have massaged the upper back and shoulders for a minute or two, move your right hand to the bottom of the neck or at the first thoracic vertebrae. Standing behind and slightly to the left of your subject, begin massaging down the back an inch or two to on either side of the spine itself. Alternate using your fingertips and the soft heel of your hand. Keep your left hand on your subject's shoulder to help support him and to balance yourself while massaging.

Use small circular motions with enough pressure that you reach the muscles under the skin. Continue this circular massaging motion along the side of the spine from the upper back down to your subject's waist. Then massage back up the same side of the spine all away up to the neck. Repeat this whole process on the side of the spine nearest you.

You may also massage along the spine itself with your fingertips, feeling your way around the vertebra with a moderate pressure. Avoid putting pressure on the ridge or the very center of the spine, but work around it. This can have a soothing, relaxing effect on your subject. Work along the spine this way or a few minutes. Then move back up the spine to the shoulders, continuing to massage along the spine.

Once more, you may knead along the shoulders with both hands. Then brace his left shoulder again with your left hand and, with the flat of your right hand, massage the upper back and along the spine again. Because your subject will be wearing a shirt, you must let off on the pressure of your hand to move it to the next area before continuing to massage, otherwise the cloth of the shirt will move with your hand.

Work your way up the back again, this time to the base of the neck. Move your left hand from your subject's shoulder to his forehead and begin massaging the back of his neck with your right hand. Do this by placing your thumb on one side of the neck and first two fingers on the other side. Use small circular motions, working your way from the base of the neck up to the base of the skull. Massage only on each side of the neck vertebra rather than on the center ridge. Make several "roundtrips" from the bottom of the neck—still on the back of the neck—up to the skull.

Then, with your left hand remaining on the forehead, make your right hand into a claw shape and begin massaging the back of the skull with your fingertips. This can be a moderately heavy massage, vibrating your fingertips into the scalp. The scalp should move with your fingertips. This massage motion is not like that of a shampoo in which you move your fingertips over the scalp in a scratching motion. This requires, instead, a heavy enough pressure to move the scalp under your fingertips.

After you have worked the back of the head, use both hands to simultaneously massage both sides of the head above the ears. Continue to use the moderate fingertip pressure and the vibrating motion massage on the scalp. Include the sides and the top of the head in this massaging. Avoid using any pressure on the temple area, i.e., between the ears and corners of the eyes.

When you have massaged the entire scalp with moderate pressure, lighten the pressure and continue the massage with a shampoo-like motion. Keep in mind that your intention is to relax your subject. Continue with this light, soothing scalp massage for another minute or so. If you can do this final minute with the idea of putting your subject to sleep, it will have a much more relaxing effect.

Finish the massage by resting your left hand on your subject's forehead and right hand on the back of his head. Sort of cradle the head between your hands for thirty seconds or so, then move your right hand down to the top of the spine and your left hand on your subject's left shoulder. Your subject should now be in the relaxed, receptive state in which you can do the suggestive magnetic treatment as described in the next chapters.

In choosing which of these relaxation methods to use for a subject, first consider his or her physical condition.

For example, if the person you are to treat is bedridden, you may be able to use only method number one, two, or three. If you are competent at, and choose to use massage, make sure your subject agrees to it and that he or she has no physical problems which might be adversely affected by massage. Never massage over any injured, healing, or diseased area of the body. When in doubt, use one of the verbal relaxing methods instead.

Because of my training and experience, I am naturally inclined to use massage along with verbal relaxation in the treatments I do. Yet, there are times when I use no massage, relying instead on verbal suggestion to relax my subject.

The method of relaxing your subject that you choose to use also depends on your preference and ability. All of these methods are to be done in an attitude of spirituality conveyed by your healing intention. Your preparation for the treatment should insure this attitude. You may use any of these relaxation methods, or a combination of any of them depending on what you feel you can do best and what would be most appropriate for your subject.

Who Should be Allowed
in the Treatment Room?

Because the healing environment is easily disrupted, it is usually best that only the healing facilitator and subject be in the treatment room. Exceptions to this policy may be allowed, however. In cases where the subject's condition is very serious, a few friends or family members may enhance the environment. They must be sincere in their concern and desire to support the healing effort.

By praying or meditating during the treatment they become involved in it. They may contribute, if they wish, by silently meditating on the affirmation which the healing facilitator uses as the verbal suggestion in the treatment. It is probably best that these people keep their eyes closed and maintain a sense of reverence and faith.

People should not be allowed to sit in on a treatment if they are merely interested or curious. And *never, never* let a skeptic attend a healing session. The treatment room should be filled with faith, hope, and expectancy. Anyone with attitudes unsupportive of the treatment must not be allowed in the room.

Personally, I find I can better perform my responsibilities as healing facilitator when there are only myself and the person receiving the treatment in the room. With no one else in the room I'm able to concentrate fully on the treatment and not be concerned with what others might think about the methods I'm using.

An alternative to having concerned relatives or friends of the subject in the treatment room is to have them pray or meditate somewhere else. You should welcome such spiritual support. It is not necessary, however, that those willing to contribute such support be physically in attendance.

The first part of the healing environment will have been established to the best of your ability when you have prepared yourself as encouraged in the last chapter, prepared the healing room atmosphere, and effectively relaxed your subject. You would then be ready to begin the magnetic healing and suggestion, the second half and the heart of the healing treatment.

6

HANDS ON

Treatment can begin when preparation, including the relaxation of your subject, is completed. Laying on of hands is done simultaneously with suggestion. Suggestions, however, are given only intermittently while magnetic healing is done for the duration of the treatment.

Up to the point where you began the magnetic healing you will have spent five to ten minutes or so getting your subject into the relaxed state. The healing treatment itself usually takes ten to twenty minutes, although occasionally, Edgar Cayce did recommend as long as an hour.

Cayce distinguishes magnetic healing from suggestion in his readings by using the former term to mean the transmitting of electromagnetic vibrations through the hands, while suggestion usually meant verbal suggestion. Sidney Weltmer, on the other hand, often used the term "magnetic healing" to mean the whole treatment, including both verbal suggestion and laying on of hands.

In his book, *The Healing Hand*, published in 1922, Weltmer wrote, "... *The whole secret of magnetic healing, including everything in it from a scientific point of view* [is]... *when I exercise a certain intention and delegate it to my hand, or have stated my intention in words that can be understood, I have used magnetic healing.*" He goes on to explain his idea of the laying on of hands: "*The best way to* [delegate your attention to your hand] *is to think, 'I will put my hand there and let it convey one healing thought for fifteen minutes.' It will take a special effort of yourself to change the intention you have delegated to your hand. That is the whole secret of the laying on of hands, and that is all the secret there is about it.*"

Weltmer spoke with a confidence that came from years of healing practice based on his spiritual philosophy. As mentioned earlier, the act of doing suggestive magnetic therapy is simple; it is the preparation that is the challenge. The simplicity of this healing method can therefore be deceptive. For without a solid foundation of understanding and preparation, the act itself is unlikely to be effective.

Why the Laying on of Hands?

If suggestion influences the subconscious to make it receptive to healing, why is it necessary to use laying on of hands at all? Indeed, suggestion can be successfully used alone. With the use of all three simultaneously, however, may there not be greater chance of healing happening?

Remember, Weltmer's method consists of three main components: intention, suggestion, and the laying on of hands. This spontaneous healing is elicited in your subject by: (1) directing the healing intention via thought from the healer's mind to her subject's mind and unconscious, (2) vocalizing the intention as suggestion or affirmation to influence the subject's subconscious, and (3) laying-on-of-hands that the vibrations raised by preparation, intention, and concentration may be transmitted by physical contact.

Actually, magnetic healing, or the laying on of hands, can do several things to encourage spontaneous healing.

Energy Transfer

First, energy, may be transmitted from healer to subject. This can result in a noticeable increase of energy in the subject. I have had people tell me after a treatment that they experienced such increased energy, yet, I felt no drain of energy myself. The validity of magnetic healing, as well as confirmation that energy transfer does take place, is noted in Edgar Cayce reading 445-2:

(Q) Is there any treatment, known today in the field of electromagnetic treatment that is superior to the physical treatments being used?

(A) *If physical electromagnetic treatments are given by those who have the ability to store within themselves those energies that may be transmitted to bodies, nothing surpasses.*

Because of this energy transfer in magnetic healing, Cayce sometimes advised that more than one person act as healing facilitator when there is the need to do a great number of treatments. Such was the case of a cancer patient whom Cayce recommended continuous treatments with only about an hour rest between sessions. In most cases, though, a subject would be given only one treatment a day, even when treatments were to be continued for weeks or more. Thus in most situations the healer will not feel fatigue after a treatment. His spiritual, mental, and physical preparation would provide him with adequate energy. Ideally, most energy transferred to the subject would not come from the healing facilitator, but from the Universal Source or God.

Though focusing is required to direct healing energy through the hands, it should not be of such intense concentration as to be stressful to the healer. There have been reports of healers perspiring profusely while giving treatments and being totally exhausted when finished. This would indicate that the healer was relying solely on his or her own energy to heal. This should never happen when giving suggestive magnetic treatments. Such strain implies that the healing facilitator is the source of healing and not God, the unlimited Creative Force.

Jump Start

Besides sending energy to the subject, magnetic healing may also provide a creative vibration that the subject can duplicate. This is similar to jump-starting a car. Once the stalled car is started, it runs on its own. Cayce refers to the need for vibrations to be "raised" within the ailing person. Of course, the atoms that compose our bodies are already vibrating. It is when these vibrations become inharmonious to health that they must be raised to restore health.

The healer, having raised his vibrations by preparing for the treatment, and by focusing on his healing intention, transmits these high vibrations by touch or laying on of hands. It is like two tuning forks with the same pitch (purpose, intent). Start one vibrating and move it close enough to the second one and it will begin the same pitch or vibration. Then move the first tuning fork away (representing the healing facilitator) and the second fork (representing the subject) continues to vibrate without the help of the first. Thus, the healer through magnetic healing seeks to awaken the Divine within the subject so that healing may occur.

The Hands Also Convey Suggestion

Weltmer concluded that, in addition to its magnetic effects, laying on of hands can serve to reinforce the verbal suggestion. For example, touch and heat from the healer's hand is felt by the subject. *"This heat from my hand is an indication that healing energy is now being transferred and is encouraging your self-healing system to respond."* This is a true statement, and your subject, in the relaxed, receptive state, does not challenge it. The statement is a suggestion that the mind receives, and the touch which is physically felt by the subject reinforces the verbal suggestion.

Not only does the hand support the verbal suggestion in this way, touch in itself conveys suggestion and is a physical extension of the attitude of the person touching. When you "reach out and touch someone," your attitude and purpose are expressed in the touch, in that the person touched interprets it consciously or unconsciously. To him it is suggestion to which he reacts emotionally, mentally, or physically. You cannot touch someone with your hand without it sending a message, albeit a subtle message.

We usually think of suggestion as verbal. But suggestion can be anything that influences a person or his unconscious, whether it be words, sight, smell, taste, touch, or telepathy. The hand, aside from its energy or vibrations, is a form of suggestion also in that its touch invokes a sense of credence to the healing treatment because of its traditional role in healing. In one situation Cayce advised that healing *"...may best be accomplished with the laying on of hands, that enables the individual, the entity, so be aided, to have* <u>*something*</u> *to hold onto that is as concrete as that it is battling with."* (281-5)

Touch in suggestive magnetic therapy suggests caring and healing. Thus, suggestion is transmitted not only verbally, but also by touch, and aid can come, *"... through a mental suggestion of therapeutics or suggestion through the hands..."* (4992-1)

More Attention on Intention

The healing intention focused in the hands of the healer is translated into vibration and transmitted via touch to the subject of the treatment. How to do this: think that your intention, your purpose for doing a treatment, is to initiate healing in your subject. Then, as you hold that thought in mind, bring your attention to your positive hand (right, if right-handed or left if left-handed.) Your thought itself is not sent through your hand. Instead, it produces a vibration that is conducted through your hand.

While the nervous system of your subject receives vibrations through your hand, produced by your intention and the friction from rubbing the hands together, his mind receives the healing intention in the words as the suggestion from you, the healer. Thus, the intention takes different routes to stimulate healing, i.e., through the voice and through touch. A third route is that of direct transference of intention from the mind of the healer to the mind of the subject as the healer concentrates. This, of course, is called telepathy, yet it is not unlike prayer for healing.

In a sense suggestive magnetic therapy approaches the mental, physical, and spiritual aspects of the subject; the intention addressing the spiritual, suggestion directed to the mental, and the laying on of hands appealing to the physical. Thus, the uniting of body, mind, and spirit in the oneness of purpose during healing treatments. Weltmer would call this "agreement" of the three aspects of the self conducive to healing. Edgar Cayce would call it being in "in harmony." Cayce said that a human being cannot have the physical, mental, and spiritual at odds with each other and expect healing. There must be harmony, agreement. Suggestive magnetic therapy attempts to induce such harmony in mind, body, and spirit, long enough for the subject's inner healing capacity to take over and sustain the creative vibration.

Major similarities between the Cayce and Weltmer methods of suggestive magnetic therapy are that both taught or recommended the intention, suggestion, and the laying on of hands.

However, noticeable differences do exist in orientation of the attention which is also reflected in wording of the suggestion.

Weltmer, though having a solid spiritual foundation, used more physically oriented intention and suggestion as reflected in these directions for treatment of constipation from Weltmer's book titled *Magnetic Healing:*

"Let the patient recline on a table on his side. Give general treatment to increase circulation. Relax the nervous system. Heat the hands and place the right-hand on the dorsal and solar plexus, the left-hand over the transverse colon, exercising the intention of throwing a current of magnetism from the right hand through the colon to the left hand, giving the suggestion that the heated hands and the magnetic current will establish proper action and cause the bowels to move freely."

This is typical of Weltmer's instructions for specific ailments. Usually he first recommended the "general treatment," discussed later in this chapter, then specific positioning of the hands. Intention most often focused on something physical happening, i.e., *"... the intention of throwing a current of magnetism..."* His worded suggestion was a verbal statement of his intention, as noted in these instructions for treating another ailment: *"...*[exercise, or focus on] *the intention of relaxing nervous tension and equalizing the circulation, and giving the suggestion that the heated hands will relax nervous tension and will equalize circulation in the arm, and that the magnetic current will allay the pain."* (*Magnetic Healing*, 1901)

This form of treatment which instructs the body to perform certain activities—*"equalize circulation in the arm..."* etc.—should be left to those healthcare professionals who thoroughly understand the structure and functions in the body. These quotes are used here to illustrate Weltmer's use of intention in suggestive magnetic therapy. I recommend that you use the Cayce spiritual focus of intention. As noted in reading 281-5: *"... use the... laying on of hands, with the affirmation that: There is being created that within the physical being, that will have such Christ Consciousness as to* *eradicate all disorder. These would require, to be sure, the laying on of the hand – the right-hand over the solar plexus center in the spine, or 9th and 10th dorsal, and the left-hand over the caecum and the transverse colon area."* This Cayce reading gives a spiritually worded suggestion (affirmation), yet includes instructions for the physical part of the treatment. The placement of the hands as he directed reflects the general rule of the right-hand on the spine and the negative hand opposite it on the healing part. Note the difference in the orientation of the Cayce and Weltmer suggestions which are a function of the healing intention.

While intention is not specifically mentioned in the Cayce reading, it is implied in the wording of the affirmation. That is, during the treatment the healing facilitator would focus on the affirmation, which Cayce gave, in addition to stating it vocally as suggestion.

Remember, the intention and resulting verbal sugges-tion are not directed at the conscious mind of your subject, but at his subconscious and the Divine healing nature within him.

The Positive Hand

Before starting magnetic healing the hands of the facilitator should be clean and dry. Clean hands are not only common courtesy but also a sanitary precaution.
Dry hands are required for the magnetic vibrations to flow freely.

The magnetically positive hand is the right hand for right-handed persons, the left for left-handed healing facilitators. The positive hand is the hand which transmits the energy. In most treatments the negative hand is used as a "stop" for the energy sent from the positive hand. In other words, when doing magnetic healing the positive hand transmits electromagnetic energy toward the negative hand. Ideally, between the two hands is the part or area of the body for which healing is sought.

Sincerity, preparation, intent, and concentration determine the quality of the vibrations and their flow to the subject of treatment. Sustaining of the healing environment rests solely on the healing facilitator after the subject has been put into the passive, relaxed state before the laying on of hands begins.

When the healer brings her attention to her hands, especially her positive hand, the energy becomes concentrated there. One may argue that the act of thinking about an area of the body only brings a heightened awareness of that part, and not any increased energy. However, the energy felt is electrical or vibratory. By concentrated thought, energy may be directed. In one of the Edgar Cayce readings discussing self-healing he supported this idea. When the vibrations are raised as in meditation, he stated, they may be directed to the ailing part simply by thought, or by mentally directing the vibrations raised to the ailing part.

To enhance the flow of energy, both Cayce and Weltmer advised that the hands be rubbed together. Friction creates heat that radiates vibration to the subject's body as explained in Cayce reading #5702-2:

(Q) Please explain just which form of electrical treatment or current, this body should have, and just how it should be applied to the body.

(A) *That current should have been applied that is of the making from the electrical forces of the body itself applying same, or electromagnetic forces, as is made by the body applying same, radiating same from its own energy of the body, and not by mechanical or by any static or creative energy outside the human body. By the storing of energy in self, and by the rubbing of hands force the body to that state wherein heat and vibration may be radiated to another body.*

Cayce refers here to magnetic healing as using energy from the healer's own body to add, "strength and vitality" to the subject. As noted earlier some healers use only their own energy. However, suggestive magnetic therapy relies less on the facilitator's energy and more on the vibrations raised in the healer's mind and transmitted through her hand.

Both Cayce and Weltmer also recommended making the hands tremble. Weltmer advised to trembling because he believed it enhanced the verbal suggestion. Cayce advised it to produce radiation, *"These are not mass-ages... but gently hold the hands in these positions. And little trembling sensation or an occasional rubbing of the hands together will produce the radiation."* (1372-1)

It would be well to note the distinction between "pure" lying on of hands, and "pure" magnetic healing. The latter is as the Cayce readings above states: the storing and using of self's energy. While in true lying on of hands, the healing facilitator is strictly a channel of the Universal Creative Energy using none of his or her own energy. Suggestive magnetic therapy combines both laying on of hands and magnetic healing. For this reason, the two terms are used synonymously throughout this book. Indeed, Cayce often did likewise in his psychic readings.

As healing facilitator, remember to rely more on God to supply the healing vibration than on self. Focus healing thoughts not only from your mind to your subject's mind, but concentrate your thoughts in your hand that these high vibrations may be conveyed through them also. In so doing you make your treatments spiritual healing experiences, appealing to the Divine nature within yourself and those you have the opportunity to aid.

Hand placement

Placement of the healer's hands depends on whether a general or specific treatment is to be done. General treatment will be used most often when the subject lacks physical or mental vitality. When the physical condition of your subject is known, either by a doctor's diagnosis or by the subject's own assessment, then treatment may be done with the hands placed with the diagnosed condition in mind.

Never take it upon yourself to diagnose your subject's condition unless you are a qualified professional. While you may treat most conditions, you must not be the one who determines what the condition is. Remember that your treatments are not substitutes for, but spiritual supplements to, medical care. When you treat specific ailments your healing intention is the same for any condition, and that is to initiate spontaneous healing within your subject. Putting your hands on a specific area of the subject's body is done so that your healing intention and electromagnetic vibrations may be directed to the part in need of healing.

Also remember that the laying on of hands is but one of three ways that suggestive magnetic therapy seeks to initiate healing within your subject. Intention is communicated mentally, verbally with suggestion, and physically through the hand. Concentration or focusing on the healing intention raises the vibrations within the healer and radiates through the positive hand. Therefore, the better you are able to keep your attention on your intention when your hands are in place, the more likely will be your success as healing facilitator.

As a general rule, the right, or positive hand is placed on the spine where the nerves exit the spinal column to various organs and areas of the body, with the left or negative hand near or over the ailing part. This is usually, but not always, the way the positive and negative hands are positioned. In a few situations Cayce advised doing the opposite—that is, place the positive hand over the ailment and the negative hand on the corresponding area of the spine. This will be discussed later.

Cayce sometimes mentioned that the healing facilitator's hands be placed directly on the subject's skin and not through their clothing. *"Place the left hand under that area almost between the shoulders and the right hand over the area where the pain and spasmodic reaction occurs at times. This would be direct to the skin, of course."* (2187-1) This reading was given for a woman with cancer. The magnetic treatments were in addition to other therapies.

Many treatments involve placing the negative hand on a part of the body that is normally not covered by clothing, i.e., the hands, arms, legs, feet, head, and neck. However, the torso is usually clothed as is the spine. Treatment with clothing between the hands and body is necessary in most cases. While this may inhibit perfect flow of the magnetic energy to the subject's body, if the clothing is lightweight and preferably only one layer, I feel that the treatment, if not as effective as hands directly on the skin, is nearly as effective. I prefer that lightweight cotton be worn by the subject, rather than man-made or synthetic fibers. While I know of no scientific basis for this, I feel that the hands radiate electromagnetic energy through this lightweight natural fiber more effectively than through synthetics.

Personally, I never concern myself with having to do treatment through clothing rather than with hands directly on the skin. I do, however, ask subjects to wear light-weight cotton if at all practical for them to do so.

The General Treatment

Sidney Weltmer advised that in most cases, the healer would not know the exact nature of the subject's ailment. In such cases, as well as for people who were simply mentally or physically fatigued, he recommended what he referred to as the "general treatment." This treatment, in Weltmer's own words, is as follows:

"A general treatment is intended for the whole physical organism, as distinct from the treatment of any special part or organ. It is intended to tone up the whole system, to equalize the nervous system, to increase or equalize the circulation of the blood, to relieve from depressed spirits or strengthen a weak physical condition.

"To give a general treatment, let the patient assume a sitting position, clothing loosened at the waistline, then, with the hands [on] the body, the right-hand on the patient's back, your left hand in front, stroke the spinal column from the cervical plexus down to the end of the spinal column, using the intention of stimulating the nervous system, increasing the circulation of the blood and giving suggestions to your patient that what you are doing will accomplish this result. Do not think the result is to be accomplished by the vigor of the stroking. *Remember, the laying on of hands or stroking is to assist the suggestion to enter the unconscious mind and accomplish the purpose intended.*"

Laying on of hands in suggestive magnetic therapy usually lasts ten to twenty minutes or more. Rather than continuous stroking, as Weltmer seems to imply here, you may use the following alternative: slowly stroke the entire spinal column several times, then hold your right hand on the cervical area (back of the neck) for a minute or so, letting the vibrations from your hand radiate into the nerves there. Next, put your right hand on the spine just below the neck at the shoulder level. Hold your hand, there for a minute or two, and then move it to the next position down the spine.

As you do the magnetic treatment, focus your mind on your healing intention. If your mind strays to irrelevant thoughts, the vibrations from your hand will change also, because your thoughts produce or influence the vibrations transmitted.

Continue this procedure of placing your positive hand on the spine—each time a hand's width lower—and after holding it there for a thirty seconds or so, move it to the next lower position. After your positive hand has rested on the last position, the sacrum, for a minute or so, end with two or three long strokes from the neck all away down the spine. See 6A on the next page.

When doing this procedure, let the palm of your positive hand, rest over the spine as in the drawing.

During this treatment you would repeat the suggestion to your subject several times, but not continuously.

Place your left hand on the front of your subject on the chest if your subject is male or, if female, just below the neck where the collarbones meet. Or you may simply rest your left hand on the shoulder of your subject. If your subject is reclining—lying face down—you may stand or sit on his or her right side, resting your left hand on the lower back or sacrum while the right hand follows the procedure described above. See figure 6B on the next page.

The Hand Vibrations

Vibrations that are transmitted by magnetic healing are usually so subtle as to be imperceptible. It is not a visible shaking of the hands. Sometimes there may be some slight feeling of electrical energy. On rare occasions a definite electrical vibration is felt. In typical suggestive magnetic treatments, vibrations from the positive hands are experienced as heat. And, while we have noted earlier that Cayce and Weltmer advised rubbing the hands together to create heat, the healer's thoughts and intention conducted through the hands generate heat as well.

Cayce has told us that atoms and cells have consciousness, and that to bring about healing they must be made aware of their Divine source. In so doing the vibrations that have become inharmonious with life-sustaining vibrations, regain their creative equilibrium.

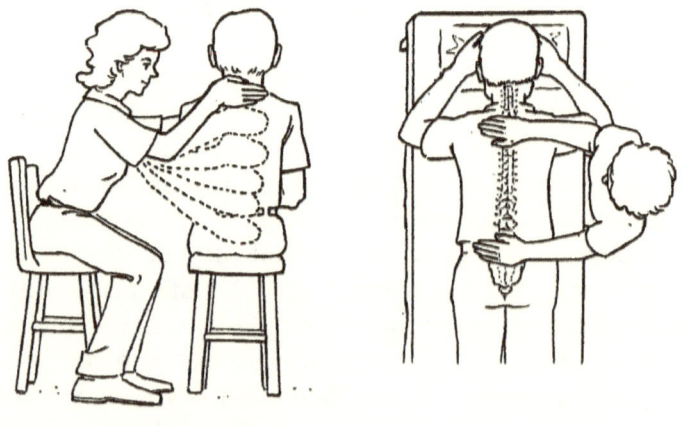

Figure 6A   Figure 6B

It is the purpose of laying on of hands to be instrumental in this renewal of life-sustaining vibrations at the cellular and atomic levels. You may remember Cayce said that God manifests in the material world as electrical vibrations. The physical body, at the cellular level, is vibrant with electrical energies. It should be no surprise then that the vibrations via the hand affect the electrical nature of the body and that the vibrations raised by prayer, meditation, and healing intention, are constructive to the physical organism.

Christ consciousness, being synonymous with God—with life itself—then, is the highest vibration. To the extent that we are able to reach and hold that creative state of consciousness do we transmit it to the subject of our treatment.

When we place our hands on the subject's body, we do so to send vibrations along the nerve routes to the ailing organ or area. This means placing the right hand or positive hand on the spine from where the nerves exit and our negative hand nearest the ailing part. There are exceptions to this rule in the Cayce readings. But, before we discuss these exceptions, we will consider the general rule first.

Treatment of Specific Ailments

Look at the drawing of the spinal column, Figure 6C. on the next page. All you need to know in order to do treatment for a specific area of the body is to know where nerves leading to it originate at the spinal cord and where the ailing part or area of the body is located. Then lightly rest your positive hand at the appropriate area on the spine and your left hand or at or near the ailing part.

For example, if you are to treat the eyes of your subject, your right hand will be on the neck (the cervical vertebra) and the base of the skull with your left hand rested over the eyes. Then you would simply keep your hands in these positions for about ten minutes or so. You may, if your intuition nudges you to do so, switch hands for part of this treatment. This, of course, is the exception to the general rule of the right or positive hand being placed on the spine. You should follow the general rule and only reverse the hand positions when your intuition strongly moves you to do so.

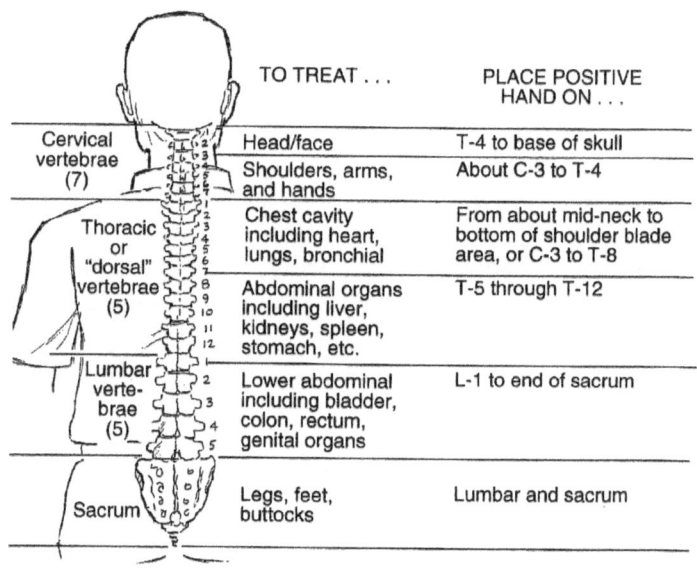

	TO TREAT . . .	PLACE POSITIVE HAND ON . . .
Cervical vertebrae (7)	Head/face	T-4 to base of skull
	Shoulders, arms, and hands	About C-3 to T-4
Thoracic or "dorsal" vertebrae (5)	Chest cavity including heart, lungs, bronchial	From about mid-neck to bottom of shoulder blade area, or C-3 to T-8
	Abdominal organs including liver, kidneys, spleen, stomach, etc.	T-5 through T-12
Lumbar verte-brae (5)	Lower abdominal including bladder, colon, rectum, genital organs	L-1 to end of sacrum
Sacrum	Legs, feet, buttocks	Lumbar and sacrum

Figure 6C

During this time while doing the magnetic healing or laying on of hands, you would repeat your suggestion or affirmation every two minutes or so. You would also concentrate on your healing intention during the whole treatment. You may end a treatment when you feel it is time. Twenty minutes is usually long enough for most treatments. Longer periods may tire both yourself and your subject. It is okay to use a clock. However, do not use a timer or the alarm on your clock. You want to bring your subject back to normal consciousness easily rather than abruptly or with a startling noise

When doing treatments for particular problems, such as the one above for the eyes, you may place your hands in specific positions. However, it is wise to always use general suggestions or affirmations rather the suggesting to the body that it respond in a certain way. Unless you are healthcare professional who thoroughly knows the body's physiology and anatomy, you should use only suggestions that are of a general healing nature. Cayce cautions against use of specific suggestions to the physical body, unless one is qualified to do so. This was Cayce's advice to one aspiring healer in reading 3068-1:

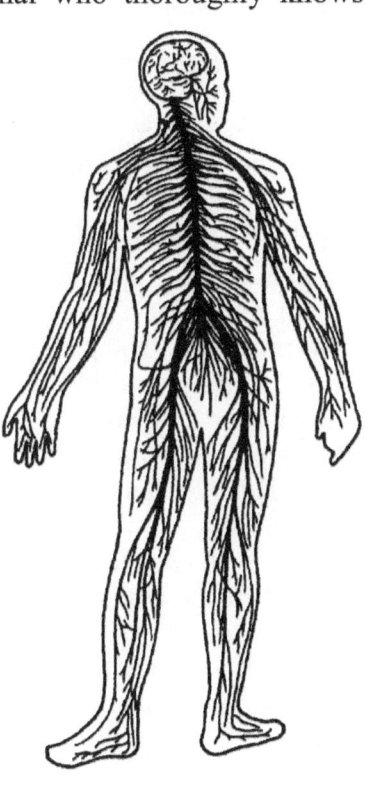

Do not attempt to use centers, segments or the structural portions, unless the body considers also that the anatomical structure of the body must be entirely understood. For, applying such would then become dangerous, unless there is full

Figure 6D

Illustration showing the profusion of nerves originating in the cerebrospinal nervous system branching out to all parts of the body.

134

comprehension, physically, mentally, spiritually of such structure, such functioning, such activities of a body.

You should, of course, use common sense when placing your negative hand at the ailing part. You would not put your hand directly on an injured or infected part when doing so might further harm it or expose yourself to disease.

More Examples of Specific Treatment

In most cases it is easy to place the positive hand on the spine and the negative hand on the ailing part. The healing facilitator will have little problem reaching the front of the body with her left (negative) hand while her right hand is in the proper location on the spine.

Take, for example, a case in which a subject is having digestive problems. The healer, sitting on the left side of her subject (who would ideally be sitting on a stool with no back support), would have no difficulty placing her right hand on the spine and left hand on her subject's abdomen. Her right hand would be on the areas from thoracic vertebra number five (T5) down to nine (T9), and possibly to L12 (see figure 6C).

Placement of the healer's left hand may be directed by the subject who would put it on the area of discomfort. The facilitator will place her right hand along the back as noted above. She may use her intuition as to the exact hand placement within the area from T5 to L2.

The subject must of course be in a passive/receptive state of consciousness before the magnetic healing and suggestion is begun. Therefore, if you needed your subject to tell you where to place your left hand you would do so before treatment begins. Otherwise, asking for such directions after treatment has begun would distract and bring the subject out of the passive state.

With hands in place, concentrate on your healing intention, and every few minutes repeat the verbal suggestion. During the ten to twenty minutes or so of the magnetic healing, you may feel that you should move your hand to slightly different positions, especially your positive hand on the spine. Your intuition may direct you, or you may sense that you should move your positive hand to make a better connection to the nerves leading to the area being treated. When this occurs, move your hand along the spine without lifting it off the back.

Remember to rub your hands together to create heat or radiation, and then dry them if necessary. You may feel that you need to rub your hands together again during the treatment. If so, do it quietly and in an easy matter so as not to distract your subject anymore than necessary. Usually you would only need to rub your hands together at the beginning of the treatment. This is because your hands, especially the positive hand, will generate heat on its own, a result of your focusing on your healing intention and directing the energy through your hand.

As most ailments are in the torso or head they can easily be reached. However, it may not be so easy to reach the lower legs or feet with your left hand while your positive hand is on the spine. In such cases, a variation of the normal treatment is required. You may, then, first place the right hand on the lower spine or sacrum to stimulate the nerves leading to the legs and feet. After resting your hand there for a few minutes, bring both hands down to the ailing part. You may then place both hands around the part and let the vibrations pass through it.

For example, if your subject has some problem with an ankle, you would first treat the lower back, and then move both hands to encircle the ankle. Place the hands directly on the ailing part—the ankle in this case—if there is no danger of harming the part you are treating.

Placement of the hands is always gentle and relaxed. No pressure is required to radiate vibration through your hand. Just the resting of hands in place is all that is necessary in magnetic healing.

Position of Your Subject

While it is usually most convenient if your subject is able to sit on a stool during treatment, sometimes it is best that he or she have treatment while lying down.

If a general treatment is to be given, the subject should be either sitting or lying face down. However, for some specific ailments Edgar Cayce advised that the subject be lying face up (supine). In such cases, the healer was instructed to reach under the subject's back to place the hand on the spine: *"Sitting upon the left side of the body (so as to make the applications easier), rub the hands well together, dry, and then place the right hand... Over the 5th and 6th dorsal center—next to the flesh itself— that is, under the spine at this area, see?"* (2474-1)

You will find that it is difficult to reach the spine with your subject lying on his or her back. One way to make this easier is to place your hand on the appropriate area of the spine while your subject is sitting up. Then, hold your hand in place as your subject lowers his or her back to the reclining position. With your hand under the back you can easily place your left hand on the ailing part on the front of the body. As this is an awkward position—your subject lying on your hand—you would only give such treatments for people who cannot lie on their side or sit up for treatment.

Use your own judgment and feedback from those you treat as to which position is best. It is easiest for you, as the healer when the subject can sit up for treatments. Your subject's comfort should take precedence, however, for he or she must be able to relax and assume a receptive state of mind for treatment to be effective.

7

SUGGESTION

—

(Q) What is the best way or method of treating her from a psychological standpoint?
(A) As of suggestion in the ordinary everyday conversation, making positive suggestion for the body. (5048-2)

In the better applications...would require...one who may subjugate through hypnosis, or through that of the power of suggestion...(5598-1)

Suggestion can come to us through any of our senses to influence our thinking or actions. For our purposes we are most concerned with the sense of hearing and suggestions which come to it from the voice.

As seen in the two readings quoted above, Edgar Cayce used the word "suggestion" in its whole range of definitions, from suggestions used in everyday conversation to that of deep hypnosis. Even in its most casual sense, suggestion can motivate, can help to change us for better or worse.

Cayce gave trance readings in deep hypnosis—probably the most extreme degree of suggestion one can experience. He was able to respond in that state to suggestions which we in our waking state cannot do. That is, he could provide intelligent information on subjects about which he knew nothing in his normal waking state.

At the other end of the spectrum of suggestions are those which we receive in our normal conversation. The family member who says, "It's a perfect day to wash the car," has no intention of doing it herself; she is suggesting, hoping someone else will volunteer to do it. She could have said, "John, go wash the car right now." However, hearing a direct command, John is likely to raise objections, resulting in an argument.

Between a hypnotic trance state and the wide awake state is the relaxed/passive state where suggestions are given in suggestive magnetic therapy. The state of consciousness your subject will be in is not one exact state. His consciousness will most probably fluctuate from that of being in the near-normal conscious condition to that of dozing off. Ideally, he would be closer to the latter state.

Reaching the Subconscious

Because it is the subconscious mind which we must influence to bring about healing, that is where we aim our suggestions. Whatever our conscious minds believe, the subconscious mind accepts as true, whether or not it is actually true. But it is our conscious mind that reasons, tries to determine what is true, and utilizes information for decision making.

When someone experiences physical challenges, such as injury or illness, the sensation of pain is a form of negative suggestion. The ailing person may also get a discouraging prognosis, adding to his doubts about his chances of recovery. Though the pain may not be a symptom of a serious problem, and whether the prognosis is accurate or not, the conscious mind may, nonetheless, fear the problem and its outcome.

For suggestion to be effective in facilitating healing it must get through these doubts and fears to reach the subject's subconscious. If we give him healing suggestion in his normal conscious state, his reaction will be to disagree, to doubt. He feels the pain, he recalls the dim prognosis, and we're telling him that his body will respond to our healing suggestions and heal itself. No matter how badly he may want to believe, there is the prognosis and the pain to make him doubt. *"Lord, I believe, help thou mine un-belief."* (Mark 9:24) He wants to believe, but can't. There's "evidence" that says he won't get well.

As long as a subject doubts suggestions that healing can happen in his body, obstacles to his healing remain. If he could just agree, believe that healing is possible, he could heal.

Sidney Weltmer's philosophy of healing and suggestive magnetic therapy was based on agreement. He considered agreement between subject and healer to be essential to healing. That is, the subject must agree with, or believe, the suggestions given by the healer for them to be accepted and acted upon by his subjective mind. As mentioned earlier it was the Bible verse Matthew 18:19 which convinced Weltmer of the healing power of agreement: *"...if two of you shall agree on earth as touching anything that they ask, it shall be done for them of my father which is in heaven."*

Now, if agreement is not forthcoming while in the normal waking state, how can we solve this? We can use the passive/receptive state of consciousness which was explained in Chapter 5. When suggestions are given while the subject is in this state, his mind will not put up objections. They pass through his conscious mind reaching his subconscious mind unchallenged.

Weltmer gave very a humorous illustration to explain what happens in this process. He related this story: During the Civil War when troops were sometimes camped near farms, orders were given forbidding the soldiers from raiding chicken coops at night to enhance their rations. A guard was posted to make sure raids did not occur. However, some of the soldiers got the idea that if they could distract the guard, they could get the chickens. It worked.

The guard, Weltmer contended, is like the conscious mind blocking our way to the subconscious. If the conscious mind is distracted, we can make our way to the subconscious without being challenged. Subliminal advertising takes the same approach. There's no need to "knock the guard out," only to distract it.

Once, after I had just finished doing a massage, my client complained about feeling nauseous. Naturally, it disturbed me to hear that my massage had made him sick when it should have been beneficial. Upon my questioning him, he said he had eaten a spaghetti dinner just before the massage. After telling him that was not such a good idea, I asked if he would allow me to try a healing technique I had recently read about. I was referring to the Sidney Weltmer method of suggestive magnetic therapy.

He agreed, and I briefly explained the technique to him. I was not very far along in my study of the method. I did not follow the exact procedure. I simply had him sit and read a newspaper comics page to get his mind occupied on something positive (humor usually has a positive effect on mind and body). I sat at his left side, placed my right hand on his spine, opposite his stomach and my left hand on his stomach. I was not yet well versed in giving verbal suggestion, so I simply focused healing thoughts toward my right hand, hoping the technique would work. Soon my client said the nausea had left him.

Possibly just having him sit for a while reading the comics alleviated the problem. Or maybe the hand magnetic energy and healing thought did it, or a combination of both. Whatever was responsible changed the vibrations in his body and resolved the nausea. I would not recommend having your subject read the comics in lieu of more relaxing methods; however, in this case I resorted to expedient means which worked to my relief as well as my client's.

Welter recommended that the subject focus on a pleasant scene or a loved one. He would then proceed to relax the subject.

When the subject is in the positive, relaxed state focusing on the positive thought, he will be in the receptive condition where suggestions can reach his inner mind. He may, if properly relaxed, drift in and out of the sleep state. That is okay. In fact, Cayce said that suggestion is most effective for children when they are dozing off—not in deep sleep, but as they drift into sleep. This may be the case for adults as well as children.

Positive Suggestions Only, Please

We learned in Chapter 5, that the healing environment should be as positive as possible. This includes the suggestion given to your subject when in the passive state. Suggestion to the subconscious mind should consist only of positive words. Rather than saying, "you are not sick," to use a simple example, you might say, "The body is healing itself now. Every atom, every cell, vibrates to the Christ consciousness." You can learn to word suggestions to suit your own spiritual preferences and do so without the use of negative words.

Henry Reed in his book titled, *Your Mind*, says that the subconscious ignores the negative words in suggestions, as it were, and accepts the remaining words. Therefore, if you were to suggest to someone in the passive state, "You no longer have the urge for cigarettes. You will not smoke." Drop the "no" and "not" and what do you have left? Just the opposite of what you desire to do. That is, you'd be reinforcing the smoking habit instead of helping to break it.

As Cayce said, *"Always [use] constructive, never negative suggestions!"* (1163-2)

(Q) Will following this treatment prevent bed wetting?
(A) This may be accomplished best by suggestion in this direction as the body is almost asleep, by the one who makes the application of the massage and rubs. Positive suggestion! Not that she won't do, but that she will do this or that, see? [Suggest] that when the desire is for the activity, the body will arouse and tend to same! (308-2)

This reading was for a ten-year-old girl. You will note that the reading mentions the massages and rubs rather than magnetic healing in which the hands sending energy do not move. When Cayce gave readings in which suggestion was advised for children, the suggestions were usually to be done when the child was retiring for the night. When massages, or rubs, were recommended, they were usually on the back, along the spine. Most likely the mother was to do the massage and the suggestion. During such massage the hands cannot help but radiate magnetic energy. As we learned in Chapter 6, both Cayce and Weltmer advised rubbing the hands together to create heat. The heat is an indication that magnetic energy is increased in the hands. Some gifted healers can generate this heat without rubbing the hands together.

Remember to always use positive suggestion with your treatments. Just as suggestion should use only positive and constructive words, so must our thoughts in healing sessions be positive also. Our thoughts are magnified during treatments and pass on as vibrations to those we seek to aid just as surely as do vibrations pass from our hands to the person we are treating.

The Wording of Suggestions

The way you word the suggestions to use during the suggestive magnetic treatments depends on whether you want to use a purely spiritual affirmation or one worded in more general terms and directed to the body's recovery. You may also use a combination of both. You should construct your suggestions so you will feel comfortable with the wording and can verbalize them with conviction and feeling. Cayce was often asked for affirmations to be used for meditation as well as suggestions for healing. He usually complied. However, at times he stated or implied that the person doing the healing treatments should word the suggestion themselves:

(Q) Please read the affirmation or suggestion that should be given when the magnetic treatments are given.
(A) That must depend a great deal upon the character, or type of individual that's to be chosen to give these treatments! They should not be said as rote, but must be said as affirmed... (5636-1)

You can learn to write your own suggestions to use in the treatments you do by studying the Cayce examples. Some that are quoted here may be such that you may decide to use them as is. Later, as you do treatments, you will become confident that you can construct your own. You may want to have your suggestion written out to have handy when giving a treatment. I usually write out the suggestion in my initial treatment for someone. Then, if I give the same person more treatments, which is usually the case, I soon have the worded suggestion memorized or have a feeling for the wording. When you can get a feel for the intention of the words, you can then say the suggestion with conviction without repeating exactly the same words each time. Suggestion is more convincing to both your subject's subconscious and to yourself when said with sincerity, faith, and from the heart.

Suggestion Examples
from the Cayce Readings

The following suggestions were for Edgar Cayce himself. They should help you better understand the basic construction of affirmations for healing.

(Q) Give word for word, the suggestion that should be given this body [Edgar Cayce] while in the subconscious state.

(A) The circulation would be so equalized as to remove the strain from all centers of the nerve as to allow the system to assimilate and secrete property those conditions necessary for normal condition of this body.

(Q) Should this suggestion be given to this body at this time?

(A) At all times when in this condition. (294-13)

This suggestion is quite general in wording. It is the kind of suggestion we might use ourselves for a person who is physically or mentally fatigued. Though Cayce was in trance state when he said that the suggestion was to be given to him, it is just as applicable for our use. As Henry Bolduc said in his book, Self Hypnosis: Creating Your Destiny, "...*effective suggestion is far more important than the depth of hypnosis. Depth has little to do with how well you can succeed...*" Indeed, it is not necessary to use hypnosis at all. Sidney Weltmer—with his three decades of working with both hypnosis and a lighter passive/receptive state used in suggestive therapeutics—concluded that the latter condition, not hypnosis, was more effective in healing *because it proved to be the more permanent.*

Here's another suggestion Cayce constructed for himself when he was obviously in good physical condition. It is one you could use in your treatments, revising it to suit yourself while retaining the basic intent. Use this affirmation for those in generally good health:

Now we find the body very good in the physical forces of same. Only that the suggestion be given at the present time:

In the equalizing of the blood in the body, this will be in such a normal manner as to cause perfect equilibrium throughout the physical structure of the body. (294-26)

Wording in the following reading is more specific. It is given here to show Cayce's ability to diagnose his own condition and to recommend treatment in the form of suggestion.

The congestion in the nerve centers and lymphatic circulation, as pertains to muscular forces in same [neuritis] produced by the bacilli as is carried in the blood of the body by the lack of perfect eliminations in the system...The suggestion to assist same would be as this:

The eliminations as created by increased circulation through the affected portions of the system will be so increased as to eliminate the conditions necessary for normal function of system, and will continue to be in a normal manner when eliminated. (294-27)

While the wording in the suggestion sounds relatively general, it is not one we would use ourselves. We do not have the ability to diagnose as Cayce did. The suggestion he gave was to remedy a specific physical condition which he could "see" in his trance state. In this case, he determined that increased circulation to the affected areas would be the proper remedy. Common sense tells us that not all physical problems would be aided by increased circulation to the ailing part. Some conditions may be worsened by increased circulation. We, as nonmedical people, just don't know enough to diagnose and prescribe.

We can, however, easily revise the suggestion to make it one we would use. Suppose a friend or family member has gotten the above diagnosis from a doctor. The doctor is treating the condition; still, your friend would like you to do suggestive magnetic therapy for him. You do not interfere with the doctor's treatment, you enhance it. Here is one way you can word the affirmation, the suggestion you give to your subject when he is in the passive-receptive state:

The circulation within this body is functioning as is necessary to resolve the concern condition. The body's self-healing system is responding in such a way as to restore it to normal and optimum health.

Wording of this suggestion, while being general, addresses the physical problem which your friend had. There is nothing in this affirmation, which would lead your friend's subconscious mind to respond in a detrimental way. Play it safe, avoid telling the physical parts of our body—the blood, organs, etc.—to respond in a particular way because doing so may be harmful.

Keep in mind that your subject's subconscious mind not only controls the functions and processes of the body, it also knows how to keep it operating normally. When something causes disease or injury to a body, it does not mean that the subconscious has forgotten how to heal the body. It means something is overriding its normal healing response. Suggestion given in suggestive magnetic therapy is done to motivate the unconscious mind to restore health. As Cayce has told us, in healing the vibrations of the atoms within the body are changed or raised to that which is of the Creative Forces. We raise our own vibrations with such resources as prayer, meditation, and focusing on our healing intention. These creative, healing vibrations, then, are contagious, so to speak, as we pass them on to the subject of our treatments.

We can raise our vibrations and pass them on with laying-on-of-hands and general suggestions/affirmations for healing, and do so knowing there is no possibility of detrimental results.

The next Cayce reading gives excellent advice for wording the suggestion in that it affirms normalcy and also provides protection against the problem returning.

(Q) What suggestion should be given to the body?
(A) That the application of those influences in the system is creating a normal balance, and will surround the body, its functioning, its activities, with those forces that will prevent the reoccurrence of the conditions that have disturbed the body and normalcy will ensue. (286-2)

The first part of the answer above, *"... the application of those influences in the system..."* refers to treatments the person was receiving. We might word the suggestion for our use as follows:

The Christ consciousness is so raised within this body as to create a normal balance and will surround the body, its functioning, its activities, with the Universal Forces that will prevent the reoccurrence of the conditions that have disturbed the body, and normalcy will ensue.

All Things Considered

You may want to consider several more factors when wording your affirmations. First is your subject, the person you are to treat. To whom will you be giving the magnetic healing and suggestions? Though he or she will be in a relaxed, receptive state of consciousness when you say the suggestions, you still want to word the suggestion to be agreeable to your subject. If he or she might take offense at a particular approach, use another.

For example, if your subject would likely respond more readily to general physical suggestions instead of spiritually worded ones, let that guide you in the wording. Or, if your subject is not Christian and might not be receptive to the word "Christ," the suggestion could easily retain its spiritual tone by using such wording as "Universal

Forces," "Creative Energies," or "God." Simply determine your subject's preference by asking *before* you begin your treatment with him or her. Of course, if your subject is a family member, you would already know this. But for those who are friends or acquaintances, you may wish to talk with them about the wording of the suggestion you are to use during the treatments.

In creating suggestions you will also need to consider what wording is comfortable for you to use. That is, you should word healing suggestions you plan to give in such a way that you can say them with sincerity and feeling. In reading 4623-2, Cayce said, *"let the body* [you, in this case] r*epeat this affirmation/suggestion, and feel in self that consciousness that this is being conducted through those applications* [treatments.]

The suggestion should be worded in such a way that it is inspiring and moving when *you* hear yourself saying it. You may find this easier to do with spiritually oriented suggestions than with more general ones. However, as you will discover, the act and process of doing suggestive magnetic treatments is inspirational in itself. When you have prepared yourself for giving treatments, you become more aware of the spiritual nature of what you are doing. It is like praying. Can you imagine praying without some feeling or emotion and reverence? The same is true in being a facilitator for healing. You are a co-worker with God in the healing process—an awesome thing to consider. When you say the affirmation to your subject, you are, in effect, talking to the Divine within that person. For it is not possible for healing to take place without God moving, without the vibrations being raised within your subject as well as yourself.

This is a case of whether your affirmation is general in wording or more spiritual. In either case, the creative, regenerative God within does the healing. Therefore, when preparing yourself for a healing treatment, you should do so with the same effort and sincerity regardless of the wording of your affirmation or suggestion.

Treating Children

Suggestion was recommended many times in the Cayce readings for children. Various forms of therapy were advised to be administered for children as they re-tired at night. Some of these therapies include the Radio-active Appliance, Wet-cell Battery, and magnetic healing. These are all of forms of low electrical vibrations, according to Cayce. In practically all of these therapies suggestion was also recommended to be used at the same time. Indeed, suggestion was recommended frequently by itself, so convinced was Cayce of its healing powers.

He strongly advised that positive thoughts be focused upon when any of these low electrical forms of therapy are used. The reason for this, according to Cayce, is that vibrations are magnified at such times. If we are thinking positive thoughts, they are magnified and vice versa if we think negative thoughts.

When treating children the positive suggestions of the healer are received by the child as he or she is dozing off. Not only can audible suggestions affect the child, the very thoughts, mood, and intention of the healer may also be received as positive or negative vibrations by the child during the magnetic healing and suggestive therapy. For this reason it is of utmost importance that the parent prepare herself, as suggested in Chapter 4, before attempting a healing session with her child.

The following is a child's reading in which suggestive magnetic therapy was recommended. It covers all the bases, telling us who is to administer the treatment, how, when, and why, and how the suggestion is to be worded.

"These manipulations, these applications of the magnetic influences in the body of the mother making the application, will quiet the body to sleep, gently, and make the general coordination throughout the system as these glands are supplying renewed energy, as the mental activities are carried on. And during such periods, in this meditation, give from the heart to the body, these suggestions—to self and to the body:

"May there be brought into physical manifestation those things and elements as necessary for the making of perfect coordination in his body, as God, the Father, through the love as shown to man in the giving of the Christ spirit into the world, creates that necessary for the best needs of this body" (512-2)

It was the mother who was told to give the treatments in practically all the readings for children in which magnetic healing and suggestion were to be administered as the child was retiring for the night.

The suggestion or affirmation should always be repeated to the child with feeling and faith. And it is as important to prepare for giving suggestive magnetic treatments to children as it is for anyone. The parent should at least take a few minutes before the treatment to focus on those things that will raise her awareness, or consciousness, to create a healing environment. In so doing she is also more apt to give the treatment and suggestions with love and conviction. Success in being a facilitator for healing will depend on attitude and approach to giving the treatments. *"Do not make same [the suggestion] as rote, or as just something to be said, but with that intense desire to be a channel of aid and help to the individual..."* (2053-2)

The effectiveness of suggestion and suggestive mag-netic therapy should not be underestimated. It is suggestion which we give our subject while in the relaxed state that must reach, and move the Divine Force within to bring about the healing sought. Cayce believed suggestion to be especially effective for children:

(Q) Would auto suggestion be beneficial to [this] *body...?*
(A) Autosuggestion is well in any case, especially of a developing mind, especially where coordination is a result of nerve disturbance, either of a functional or mental disorder. (758-25)

Autosuggestion as the term is used today means self-suggestion. However, the above reading meant sugges-tion by the healing facilitator as the child was in the early stages of sleep.

You can enhance the feeling and sincerity you put into the treatment suggestion given to your child if you word the suggestion yourself. You may take examples of suggestion from the Cayce readings for children and reword them, keeping in mind the child's best interest when doing so. *"Not as a mother desires, but that the mother's mind be as one with the purpose for which the entity...is experiencing these conditions; and that there be fulfilled within the body and the mind for which its entrance is being experienced."* (1371-2)

Quoted below are several more suggestions Cayce gave for children. Revise them as you wish, while keeping the basic content.

As you (calling the child by its own name...) *as you sink into a quiet, restful sleep, the organs of the body will so function that the very best will be builded in the physical and mental being, giving that response that will be a normal activity for the organs of the sensory system.* (2253-2)

The body is performing its normal functioning-proper. The mental and physical well-being is coordinating in a proper manner, and will continue to do so until the body is well and strong and capable of resistance in every normal matter. (758-25)

The following reading was for an abnormal child and appeals to her spiritual nature as well as to the physical:

"May there be created through the Divine Forces in this body that which will make for the nearer and nearer normal reaction: That there may be those proper reactions for the system, that it may be a useful, self-sustaining entity." (1104-2)

When giving treatments for children Cayce advised, *"Do not continue for long periods, but two, three, four days, and then give these an opportunity then to react upon the system, see?"* (1163-2) In other words, do the treatment for a few days and leave off for several days before resuming. This gives the child's body time to respond or react to the therapy. It also will give the mother's body time to rebuild its own energy reserves.

Remember, in all treatments, whether for children or adults, the suggestion or affirmation is given while the subject is in the passive state of consciousness, and while the laying on of hands is being done. Most treatments usually last ten to twenty minutes. During that time the suggestion would be repeated every two minutes or so.

8

Review

———

Use this chapter as your guide to the suggestive magnetic therapy procedure. It is not a substitute for the more
in-depth coverage of the healing method detailed earlier,
as this review will make little sense to anyone not having
read and understood the previous chapters. However, it
can serve as a quick reference when there has been a time
lapse of a week or more between treatments. At times I
go back and review the basics of the healing method to
make sure I have not strayed from or forgotten some
important point.

An even more concise review in the form of a checklist
is featured on the last page of this chapter.

Preparation

Prepare with prayer, meditation and other ways you find meaningful before doing a treatment. This devotional is for the purpose of attunement—connecting with God—that you may go into the treatment session with a consciousness conducive to healing. Try to do this preparation at least several hours before the treatment. It would even be well to do it the day or night before a period session. I find a noticeable difference in treatments I do when I have prayed, meditated, and thought about them beforehand.

Eat sensibly the day before you are to give the treatment. Do not overeat or indulge in junk food. If possible, let two or three hours lapse between meals and the treatment session. The same holds true for the person receiving treatment. You, as healing facilitator, should advise your subject regarding this.

You may also wish to try fasting, or skip a meal or two to see if it enhances your performance as a healer. Remember, however, that the facilitating of suggestive magnetic therapy will use some of your own energy. Keep as physically fit as possible so that your energy level will be high for treatments.

The affirmation you use as the verbal suggestion during the treatment should be discussed with your subject and written before the session. Although treatments are often repeated, some many times for the same person, you need to construct the affirmation only once for the first session. Of course, the affirmation may be changed at any time that both facilitator and subject agree. In any event, you should begin treatments with the affirmation already constructed. You do not want to make a habit of reading the suggestion to your subject. But it is a good idea to write it out and have it where you can see it during treatments. Later you can rephrase it if need be.

The Treatment Room

Check out the room in which you will do the treatment. It should be quiet and in a place where you won't be interrupted. Use a room with no phone or turn your cell phones off. Appropriate music can help your subject become more relaxed and receptive to the treatment. Use music both you and your subject find inspiring and relaxing. It is best to use music with no vocals.

Ideally, your subject should sit on a stool so that you can easily reach his back and spine. However, your subject's physical condition will dictate whether he should sit or lie down. If he must lie down, have him lie face down, if possible, or on his right side. Lying face up is the most relaxing, but with your subject in that position it is difficult for you to reach his spine.

Use an air freshener only if there are offensive smells in the room. Do not overpower the room with artificial scents. Fresh, fragrant flowers such as roses may add to the healing environment.

Don't be too concerned with the visual appearance of the room. Your subject should have his eyes closed during the treatment, and you should be actively involved in the role as healer so as to be indifferent to the room's appearance. However, common sense would tell you not to use a room that is depressing. The overall feeling of the room should be positive.

Allow others in the treatment room *only* if they are in complete agreement with the healing method. Anyone sitting in on the healing session must contribute by meditating or praying for the health of the subject. No casual or curious spectators should be admitted. Skeptics are not welcome. Do not allow others into the treatment room when their presence would inhibit your role as healer.

Remember, it is of utmost importance that you do not bring any anger or ill will into a treatment. Any conscious negative attitudes should be addressed in your preparation—in your prayers and meditation. If you have any resentment or ill will toward the person seeking healing, it must be resolved before the treatment. Such attitudes must be eliminated or at least suspended for the duration of the treatment, otherwise, the treatment should be canceled. In one instance, noted in an earlier chapter, Cayce advised against a mother doing treatments for her child because of resentments between them. Doing treatments while harboring negative attitudes and emotions can cause harm rather than healing. Bring only goodwill and constructive thoughts into healing sessions, because you must be able to maintain a healing intention for the duration of every treatment.

Pretreatment Meditation

Take a minute or two just before beginning a treatment to prepare one last time. Pray and meditate, as you did earlier, this time do so to center yourself and focus on the treatment at hand. This meditation will also relax you physically so that you may turn your full attention to doing the treatment. Your relaxed state will help your subject relax, too. Include a prayer of protection that nothing negative will intrude or disrupt the treatment. Both you and the subject of the treatment may meditate together if you are comfortable with the idea. However, this pre-treatment attunement is more important to the healer. For, as treatment begins, the subject will have the opportunity to relax, even meditate, if he so desires, while you, as the healing facilitator must then become active.

These minutes of prayer, meditation, just prior to the session is an invaluable aid to enhancing your healing state of consciousness. Include it before every treatment.

Relaxing Your Subject

According to Sidney Weltmer, the success of suggestive magnetic treatments depends to a large part on the passivity of the subject. Without this relaxed, receptive mental and physical state, the suggestions given during treatment may be challenged or doubted by his conscious, reasoning mind.

You may talk your subject into the relaxed state. This is the relaxation method you should rely on most. Tell your subject that all tension is being drained out of his or her muscles. Begin with the muscles of the head, and verbally work your way down through all the muscle groups until you've relaxed the feet. Take your time and talk in a relaxed soothing matter. Tell your subject to visualize some peaceful nature scene from his or her past, or you may verbally construct such a scene. Continue to verbally relax your subject until you sense that he or she is passive, receptive, and ready for the magnetic healing and suggestion/affirmation.

If your subject is an experienced meditator he or she may use meditation for self-relaxation. Massage may also be used to relax your subject, but only if you are competent at doing massage.

Be patient and relaxed yourself while putting your subject into a relaxed state. Do not rush into doing the magnetic healing and suggestion. Wait until you are sure your subject is completely passive, for this relaxed state may be as responsible in creating the healing environment as is the treatment itself. Ideally this relaxed, passive consciousness is, or is close to, dosing. In some cases, especially with children, dosing is the preferred condition for treatment, according to Cayce.

Magnetic Healing

Begin the laying on of hands after your subject is completely relaxed. Make sure your hands are clean and dry. Rub your hands together to generate heat and better radiate healing energy. For treatment of specific ailments, find the appropriate area on the spine to place your positive (right) hand for the condition you are to treat. Your positive hand radiates energy into the nerves branching from the spine and ending in the organs or other areas of the body being treated. Position your left hand on or near the ailing part.

When doing a general treatment with your subject sitting, you may rest your left hand on his or her shoulder while placing the right hand on various positions on the spine.

For specific ailments keep your hands still for ten to fifteen minutes. Because your hands must remain in one position for so long, you must position your body— whether you are to sit or stand—in such a way that you will not become tired or cramped. Your hands and arms should stay relaxed. Energy will flow through them naturally if you will simply concentrate on your healing intention.

Intention

Your powers of concentration are tested in giving treatments. Healing with suggestive magnetic therapy requires that your mind stay on your healing intention. All extraneous, irrelevant thoughts must be kept outside. If you find your mind wandering, simply refocus on your intention. It may help to look at the affirmation that you have written and placed where you can easily see it.

Know that your healing intention is translated into electromagnetic energy. This energy stimulates nerves that provide impulses throughout the body. Its vibration also directly influences the electrical nature of the atoms and cells of an ailing part.

Your healing intention reaches the unconscious of your subject by way of the nervous system to initiate self-healing within the body. The raising of your consciousness by preparation, intention, and consideration of the electrical nature of God produces the healing vibration. This vibration, radiated through the healer's hand and mind, seek to jump-start the healing process within the person seeking healing.

Suggestion

The affirmation should be printed in large enough letters that you can read it from a few feet away. Place it where you can see it when doing the magnetic healing. Ideally you would memorize the affirmation, then para-phrase it when repeating it, being sure to keep the basic intent intact.

Give the suggestion when you've finished relaxing your subject and begin the laying on of hands. This verbal suggestion is simply the affirmation spoken aloud. You will usually do the magnetic healing for ten or twenty minutes or so. Repeat the suggestion every two or three minutes during this time. During the quiet times— between repeating the suggestion—you should con-centrate, focusing on your healing intention. You may accomplish this in a number of ways: by silently repeating the affirmation in your mind, by "seeing, feeling, and knowing" that the energy of your hands is going to the part in need of healing, or even by repeating the Lord's Prayer, etc.

Repeat the suggestion with conviction, sincerity, and belief. Say it calmly in your normal speaking voice, or lower. Avoid raising your voice as this may bring your subject out of his relaxed state.

Remember, when you repeat the suggestion you are talking to your subject's inner mind, his subconscious. His conscious reasoning mind must be relaxed and passive so that the verbal suggestion can reach his unconscious unchallenged. Suggestion, accepted by the unconscious mind of your subject, activates the re-generating, healing action of the Creator within your subject. Your job is to help this happen.

Finishing Up

Plan your treatment to last ten minutes to half an hour. Use a clock if you wish, but do not use the alarm. End the treatments by gently bringing your subject back from his relaxed state to a normal, alert consciousness. Don't startle your subject back to the here and now. If your subject is to drive or do some other activity that requires mental alertness, make sure he or she is wide awake and alert before doing so.

If your subject can continue to rest, even sleep, or nap after the treatment, so much the better. Remember, Cayce often advised that healing treatments for children be done as they are retiring for the night. When drifting into sleep, the mind is most receptive to suggestion.

After the Treatment

After you've done your best, let go and leave the results to God. Your role as healing facilitator is to initiate, to motivate the healing process within the person you are to treat. When you've completed the treatment, it is a good idea to drop the role as healer. In other words, don't concern yourself with the outcome of treatments.

As Cayce advised one mother giving treatments to her child, do the treatments for four days, then discontinue them for three. This "time off" gives the body time to absorb what was done in the treatments and to respond to them. Of course, this regimen of four days of treatments and three days off is not meant to be a rule to follow. Rather, it indicates that the body continues to react to treatment after the session ends. Indeed, if we remember that our role as healer is to initiate or jump-start self healing within the subject, you can better appreciate the healing that occurs between treatments.

A recent television show documented the story of a young woman injured in an accident. For over two months she lay in a hospital in great pain with no hope of relief or recovery. Yet, her mother prayed daily for the daughter's healing. No progress seemed forthcoming. Then one day when no one was in her hospital room, the young woman felt what she described as the pain just draining down and out of her body. Beginning at her head it moved down her body as if she were being emptied of her pain. It was over quickly. She was completely free of her condition and soon was released from the hospital. Healing—this spontaneous remission—evidently came from the cumulative effect of the mother's prayers. And it came, not when people were in her room, but when the patient was alone and unsuspecting of a miracle.

You are privileged to be a co-worker with the creative energy of the universe—God. Do not be concerned with results. Give every treatment your best effort and intentions, *and leave the results to God.*

Suggestive Magnetic Therapy
Procedure Checklist

PRIOR TO THE TREATMENT SESSION:
1) Prepare several hours before or the day before a treatment is to be given. Include prayer, meditation, contemplating God.
2) Write the affirmation to be used as the suggestion.
3) Arrange the treatment room; include relaxing music.
4) Pray and meditate again for a minute or two just prior to beginning the treatment.

THE TREATMENT ITSELF:
4) Relax your subject. Start the magnetic healing and suggestion only after your subject is completely relaxed.
5) Concentrate on the healing intention throughout the treatment.
6) Begin the magnetic healing—laying on of hands.
7) Verbally repeat the affirmation every two or three minutes.

POST-TREATMENT:
8) When finished, gently bring your subject back to normal, alert consciousness, or let him or her sleep if possible.
9) Don't concern yourself with results. Let it go and leave the results to God.

And always remember:

Suggestive magnetic therapy is NOT a substitute for proper medical care.

9

Where to Begin

———

Begin where you are—among family and friends. Again and again Cayce said that healing should and could be done by those close to us. Others may have more skill, but close associates are able to provide caring that professionals cannot. The following Cayce reading gives great insight, instruction, and inspiration for healing within a particular marital relationship:

And the hand therapy [magnetic healing]... this would <u>not</u> be done by the same person – that is, not by the [particular doctor] who corrects purely by mechanical means. For this, the hand therapy must be done in love, in harmony, in the desire for the help, with the proper reactions in the body itself.

... Let the wife rub her hands together first and then make the hand therapy application; putting the right hand between the shoulder blades on the spine, at the 3rd dorsal—or 3rd and 2nd dorsal plexus, and the left-hand over the vocal box. Let them remain this way for at least twenty minutes—just holding the right hand over that area on the spine, and the left-hand over the vocal box.

If the body can be persuaded to sleep after the first few times, much the better.

But use this period for prayer, for meditation – both the self and the wife who would be making the application of the electrotherapy of the body-emotions; for this is the entity who must forgive, if the karmic forces would be met. (2705-1)

The ability to facilitate healing has nothing to do with titles, degrees, formal or professional training. One need not be an ordained minister or healthcare professional to be a healer. Being a facilitator for healing simply has to do with understanding the healing process.

We would do these [various treatments] *with greater prayer, and the application of the hands of one so closely affiliated with the entity in its material activity.* (1936-1)

Patience and Persistence

Because treatments are not only to be done with caring, but also with consistency and persistency, often over long periods of time, it is even more logical that family or close friends act as healing facilitators. *"Be consistent, be persistent, most of all be prayerful."* (3049-2)

While some minor ailments may respond almost immediately to treatment, others may require long-term therapy. Many serious and chronic conditions require such commitment:

(Q) How much longer will [the therapies] *take?*
(A) If it's a day or a year, what's the difference if it's accomplished? There is no time! If thou art weary in that thou art doing, then turned back! (281-5)

For such serious or chronic problems which may require long-term commitment, family or other close associates would best serve as healers for several reasons. First and foremost is that family or friends are more likely to have a caring attitude. Then, too, it will be more convenient since close associates would be available to do treatments daily or frequently and at odd hours, such as at night. And because the role of healing facilitator can be assumed by most anyone, two or more members of a family could alternate as healers. Finally, any professionally healer would charge a fee or at least ask for donations for such services, which, in the case of ongoing treatments could amount to a considerable sum.

Healers as Laypeople or Professionals

Suggestive magnetic therapy, as presented in this book, is not intended to make one a professional healer who would charge for such treatments. However, where no close associates are available, willing, or suitable to do these treatments, then such a healer may be sought. Even in these cases, in light of the many variables, subjectivity, and the spiritual approach presented here, it would seem unethical to charge a fee for suggestive magnetic therapy.

On the other hand, healthcare professionals, including massage therapists may wish to include magnetic healing and suggestion in their work. That is, incorporate suggestion and magnetic therapy—or aspects of the therapy into their healing modality.

Aside from these exceptions, it is the hope of the author and purpose of this book that suggestive magnetic therapy be used by family and friends with no charge or donations accepted. For in the final analysis, treatments may be as beneficial to the healer in his or her spiritual development as it is physically to those receiving treatments.

Taking the Mystery Out of Healing

The better we understand how suggestive magnetic treatments elicit healing, the less we will regard spiritual healing as a mystery.

Keep in mind when giving treatments just what magnetic healing and suggestion do to initiate spontaneous healing in a person. Remember, also, that while proficiency at suggestive magnetic therapy comes with attitude and experience, the physical and mental equipment required to facilitate healing is inherent in us all. Thus, we should never regard "healers" with awe, but direct such regard to that healing energy, God, who does the actual healing.

The great mystery in healing is the existence of this life force rather than our ability to cooperate and work with it as healing facilitators. By understanding how suggestive magnetic therapy works, we remove the mystery from the healing process and, instead, direct our wonder to this healing vibration that pervades the universe.

What to Treat

If you are fortunate enough not to have family members or close friends with major physical problems, you will still likely have plenty of opportunity to practice suggestive magnetic therapy.

Garden variety ailments such as bumps, bruises, minor injuries, headaches, stomach distresses, and general fatigue are just a few of the ailment, which sooner or later will occur. You might even consider treating plants and pets, although their anatomy is different, they may, nonetheless, respond to your healing efforts.

These are all subject to the healing potential of your treatments. This does not preclude seeing a doctor when problems warrant it. Even when health issues require a doctor's attention, suggestive magnetic therapy can still be important. Remember that suggestive magnetic therapy is not a substitute for medical care—rather, it can serve to enhance that care even in very serious conditions. Indeed, in cases where doctors can offer no hope of recovery, spiritual healing may be one alternative that can help.

So this healing method may be used in the whole range of physical ailments from the trivial to the terminal. Of course, you must use common sense when offering to do treatments. Avoid situations that would endanger your own health, such as contagious diseases. Also, in some situations an ailing person may not be able to tolerate even the moderate touch employed in suggestive magnetic therapy.

This noninvasive and spiritually oriented therapy would be welcomed by most ailing friends and family members. Yet, you may need to be tactful when offering treatments.

Making Yourself Available as "Healer"

If you have a close-knit family and friends who have confidence in you, you should have little trouble in using suggestive magnetic therapy to help them when the opportunity arises.

Explain to them the basics of suggestive magnetic therapy, and that it may bring relief and healing or speed up the healing process. But never do a hard-sell or try to argue them into agreeing to have a treatment. That would be counter-productive and throw up barriers to healing with this healing therapy.

You may also wish to differentiate between faith healing and suggestive magnetic therapy by explaining that the former seeks instant healing, while the latter is a therapy which will require at least a half-hour session, and even ongoing treatments in the case of serious or chronic ailments.

Remember that your subject must desire healing. For without such desire, even if he should allow you to give him treatments, efforts will not likely motivate his unconscious to accept healing. Edgar Cayce was emphatic on this point. When asked by a healer which of her four healing gifts she should use to heal a certain person, he replied:

There must be the desire on the part of Carrie...to be healed! You cannot create them, no matter what thou hast! God cannot save a man that would not be saved! (281-3)

As eager as you may be to help people, your offer of treatments may be rejected by some. Your offer to treat with suggestive magnetic therapy must be welcomed if you are to create the constructive environment required for healing. There must be agreement, as Sidney Weltmer would say, or harmony between healer and subject. Do not be hurt or offended, and above all, do not be resentful of those who refuse your offer to treat them. Maintain your confidence and openness, and direct your energy to the treatments you are privileged to do. Those you help will be your best testimonial and reference.

Unless you have family members or friends with serious physical problems you may not have regular opportunities to practice. Weeks or months may go by without such an opportunity being forthcoming. Consider it a blessing if such is the case! However, when there is a time lapse of many weeks between treatments you would do well to review the healing process and procedures (see Chapter 8).

Sooner or later your healing skills will be needed and welcomed. Begin where you are and give yourself time to improve your abilities through practice. As you become more proficient, more opportunities for you to help others will likely present themselves. Be willing, also to share your knowledge of suggestive magnetic therapy with those interested. For we are all born with the potential to heal others. Nevertheless, we are all at various levels of spiritual development which may determine how effectively we are able to facilitate healing.

When You are in Need of Healing

You may now or in the future have a need for healing yourself. How do you go about finding someone to act as healing facilitator for you?

Choose favorite family members or friends in good health and with plenty of energy, who are willing to learn this healing method. Depending on the nature and seriousness of your ailment, they may need to commit time on a regular basis to do the treatments. This does not mean that the therapy must be done every day. But, with serious conditions not many days should elapse between treatments.

You may even be fortunate enough to have more than one person willing to learn and do the treatments for you. In that case they could share the responsibility and opportunity to do the treatments.

You may recall the Cayce reading in which he recommended that the chosen healer be someone whom the ailing person had helped in the past. This is an interesting statement! For what he appears to be telling us is that those we have helped in the past make the best healing facilitators for us. Is it because we "go to heaven" leaning, so to speak, on those we have helped? You should find such people—those you have helped— willing and honored to facilitate your treatments, just as you would be if some friends or relatives asked you to take on the role of healer for them.

Therefore, share this book and your understanding with like-minded people. In so doing you open opportunities of healing for both your friends and family as well as yourself.

Healing More Than Physical

The practice of healing among friends, relatives, and spouses may aid not only the physical, but current inter-personal relationships as well as what may be karmic ties. Thus, your offer to do treatments with those you have strained relationships with may help heal wounds. This does not negate the necessity to do suggestive magnetic treatments with good-will intent. Though relations may be strained, preparation with prayer and meditation can help us to do treatments with a positive and healing frame of mind. The following Cayce readings gives us more specific advice:

... First there must be a change in the mental attitude of the body. There must be eradicated that of any judgment or condemnation on the part of self, as respecting self or any associated with the body in any manner, either previously or in the present. This must be eradicated from the mind. How? By filling same with constructive loving influence toward self, toward others, and as these are raised within the consciousness of self by the proper thinking, with the less and less of condemnation to anyone, these create the proper surroundings, the proper attitude. (631-6)

I am reminded of an experience from years ago when I taught simple head-and-shoulder massage to conference attendees. In one of the workshops was a young couple, married only a few months. As usual, participants enjoyed learning and receiving the massage, and it was not unusual for them to express how much they enjoyed it. But this young married couple evidently benefited more than most. For, several months later I received some welcome feedback. Edgar Cayce's grandson had given a talk in the out-of-town city where this young couple lived. They told him that my simple head and shoulders massage workshop helped strengthen their marriage which, unbeknownst to me, and not been on solid footing when they attended my workshop. This simple massage was an opportunity for the couple to relate in an uncommon, caring way. If such a positive effect can occur by learning and practicing something as simple as head-and-shoulder massage, how much more might be act of doing suggestive magnetic therapy mend relationships?

Parents and Children

Parents have a special opportunity to help their children with suggestive magnetic therapy. This is particularly true with young children. Not only may they be more receptive to parents healing efforts, but they may be best helped while in their formative years.

You may recall from earlier chapters that Cayce advised parents—mothers especially—that bedtime is the ideal time to give healing treatments for children. At such times the relaxation procedures discussed in Chapter 5 may not be necessary if the child falls asleep easily. Then the parent may spend as little as ten minutes doing magnetic healing and suggestion.

Souls choose their parents according to Edgar Cayce. Yet, it is the parent's responsibility to help their children through difficult conditions. The following excerpt from a Cayce reading given for a child with speech impairment supports this claim.

[Helping the child], *we would say is the work if those who brought this body to this plane, that is the parents, both working in conjunction one with the other for the development of the soul of the body* [4469]*; the father and the mother together with the forces they called into themselves from the One above.*

... the forces that are to be supplied in its development are those that were not added during the normal gestation, and they must be added by the souls of the parents...one to apply through the waking state, and one in the sleep state, and through suggestion to the cellular force to carry suggestion to the whole body. These will be varied from time to time, but they must produce in the physical body the love...necessary to reproduce in itself. Do that, and we will bring through, with tedious force, a

being above the normal in its soul and spiritual develop-ment. (4469-1)

Reading and studying suggestive magnetic therapy is one thing, experiencing, giving treatments is quite another. For it can open a whole new arena of spiritual involvement and enrichment for those you are privileged to treat as well as yourself. Be patient as you develop your ability to facilitate healing. And always give credit for healing to God, the healing energy that pervades all of life that is life itself. For, *"...in him we live, and move, and have our being."* (Acts 17:28)

For Health Care Professionals
and Massage Therapists

––––––

While this book is specifically for the layperson, Cayce also recommended that massage therapists and healthcare professionals—especially osteopaths, but also others— use magnetic healing for some people who received psychic readings from him.

Healthcare professionals and massage therapists, however, may not be able to do suggestive magnetic therapy with the spiritual emphasis that a patient's family or friends would do. This is especially true regarding the wording of the suggestion or affirmation to be used in treatments. This is not to imply that either spiritually worded suggestions, or the physically specific ones are best or most effective in suggestive magnetic therapy. Which of the two is most conducive to healing most likely depends on the healing facilitator and the client or patient.

In Chapter 7 on "Suggestion," many examples of spiritually worded suggestions are given. These so-worded suggestions were typical of those Edgar Cayce gave to be used mainly by family members or associates in healing treatments. This was because the layperson usually does not have enough knowledge of physiology and anatomy to give a body specific directions for its recovery. You may recall from Chapter 6 the Cayce reading (3368-1) that warned, *"Do not attempt to use centers, segments or the structural portions,"* in giving treatments, unless one entirely understands the body, its anatomy, and functions.

Weltmer's General Treatment

Sidney Weltmer advised that the magnetic healer would not usually know, nor be in a position to diagnose, the true or exact nature of his client's physical problem. He therefore recommended what he called the "general treatment," for most cases. Weltmer's directions for doing this treatment are quoted in Chapter 6. If you refer back to this, you will see that the general treatment is simply massage along the whole length of the spine.

However, this general treatment differs from a regular back massage in that it is not a deep or heavy pressure, and it's concentrated along and beside the spine. Its purpose is to affect the nerves, not the muscles. Also, more time is taken in the magnetic treatment than in a regular massage.

Bear in mind that the healing intention and the giving of verbal suggestions are included in the general treatment, as they are in all suggestive magnetic treatments.

In addition to using the general treatment or what might be called a general physical "tune-up," Weltmer usually recommended that it precede most treatments for specific problems.

Cayce sometimes, but not always, advised having a massage prior to the magnetic treatment. In many cases he simply stated where the facilitator's hands should be placed for healing without any mention of massage.

Physically Specific Suggestions

Healthcare professionals, or massage therapists may confidently use the physically specific style of suggestion such as Weltmer used and taught. The following are typical instructions from Weltmer's writing for a specific ailment (tumors):

"Give general treatment to increase and equalize circulation, and rub gently in every direction from the tumor to stimulate the venous circulation and produce a normal condition of all the excretory organs. Instruct the patient (and insist upon close observance of your instructions) to begin and practice deep breathing for the purpose of oxygenating and producing blood; after which place the heated hand over the nerve center supplying nutrient to the part of the body in which the tumor is situated, exercising the intention to stimulate arterial and venous circulation for the purpose of carrying off and distributing the foreign substance which has accumulated and which constitutes the tumor, distributing it into the circulation, and carrying it through the excretory organs

to the outside world." (From *The Mystery Revealed* by Sidney Weltmer, 1901)

Weltmer's instructions may not be consistent with current medical knowledge. I quote this only to illustrate the detail that may be used in specific suggestions given in healing treatments. Healthcare professionals should word the suggestions they formulate from their own knowledge and training. Remember, suggestion is given to the patient on the premise that the unconscious mind will act on directions given it regarding the physical body. This is why it is important that specific suggestions be only used by knowledgeable professionals. Not all of the suggestions Cayce gave for use during magnetic healing were spiritually or even generally worded. This reading for a person with kidney problems calls for a physically specific suggestion, but leaves the actual wording of the suggestion to the healing facilitator:

With the mental force give the suggestion of action of these organs, centers and their function and connection sympathetically and organically to function properly. (Cayce reading # 4772-1)

Massage Therapy and
Suggestive Magnetic Healing

Massage therapists may have the ideal situation in which magnetic healing and suggestion can be employed. And because the massage therapist's work involves touching, he or she should be a natural for the laying on of hands or magnetic healing.

Curriculum in massage schools includes courses in anatomy and physiology, making a licensed massage therapist quite familiar with the spine and nerves leading from it. This knowledge is most helpful for magnetic healing as a positive hand is usually placed on the spine where nerves branch out and go to the various parts of the body (see figure 6D). Knowledge of the location of organs and other anatomy is necessary for placement of the left or negative hand.

The study of physiology familiarizes the therapist with the functions of organs, other structures, and fluids of the body. Such knowledge makes the massage therapist more adapt at constructing the wording of suggestions for specific physical ailments; that is, formulating the suggestions that encourage proper functioning of organs and the rest of the body. He must, of course, use discretion in doing so as he is not qualified to diagnose medical problems and prescribe treatments for them. It would be a good arrangement for massage therapists doing magnetic healing to work with healthcare professionals who are so qualified. With diagnosis and recommendations from a doctor, the therapist could give his client the proper suggestion, formulated to help heal specific conditions. Doctors who practice holistic healing might even consider writing out the suggestion to be used by the therapists giving treatments, much like a doctor would write out a prescription, except, one hopes, more legible!

Using Magnetic Healing After Massage

The most logical time for the massage therapist to use suggestive magnetic therapy is at the end of a massage as noted in reading 5307-1 by Edgar Cayce:

[The problems] *as we find are from weaknesses which have existed from a great strain put on this body through the umbilical centers. These would respond the more normally from fume baths with a gentle massage and then the magnetic treatments.*

The magnetic treatments would be right hand placed over 9th dorsal and the left hand over the umbilical center, or to the upper portion of the umbilical center. These magnetic treatments would be given daily for a period sufficient to remove these tensions and to the correct vibrations for the unison of activity of the organs of the body of the central nervous system.

...The fume baths... and then the massage with the gentle oil treatments, using peanut oil for this, and massage along the spine, not attempting to make corrections, but sufficient for the cerebrospinal centers and the sympathetic nervous system and centers to retain or gain the virility from the strengthening influence of the oils, and with the magnetic treatments bring better conditions for the body.

There are two practical reasons for doing the magnetic healing *after* the massage. First, and foremost, as a prerequisite to receiving suggestive magnetic therapy, the subject must be put in a relaxed, receptive physical and mental state, which is the usual result of a good massage. In fact, it is not uncommon for a person to fall asleep during the massage.

Second, because the therapist will have been working with his hands throughout the massage, at the end of a massage his hands would likely radiate electromagnetic energy more strongly than at the beginning. He should remember, however, to dry his hands before beginning the magnetic healing. Rubbing of the hands together again after drying them will intensify the electromagnetic energy there. It would make sense for the therapist also to remove any dampness from his client's body where he is to place his hands for healing. The therapist should do this in such a way so as not to startle his client out of his relaxed state.

Cayce stated in some of his readings on magnetic healing that the hands be placed directly on the skin and not through clothing. This presents no problem for the massage therapist who works directly on the body and not through clothing.

Massage Time Advantage

Massage therapists have a time advantage over most other healthcare professionals. Thirty minutes or an hour are standard time lengths for massage. Most therapists also do hour-and-a-half massages at proportionally higher rates. The usual time of suggestive magnetic treatments, runs from twenty minutes to half an hour, although in some cases Cayce advised longer times. In Weltmer's treatments up to half of the treatment time was used to relax the patient. Thus, in a twenty-minute treatment approximately ten minutes might be used for relaxing and the other ten for the treatment itself, i.e., the laying on of hands, and suggestion. The massage therapist could set aside ten minutes of a standard massage for suggestive magnetic therapy without increase in his or her fees. Since massage is physically more demanding than magnetic healing, it makes no sense to charge more to substitute ten minutes of magnetic healing for ten minutes of massage time.

However, the facilitating of magnetic healing is mentally and spiritually more demanding massage. So, while the therapist would do little physical work during the suggestive magnetic therapy, he or she is, on the other hand, required to be more mentally focused than when doing massage.

Healing Attitude

While positive, healing intention is an absolute necessity in suggestive magnetic therapy, it should also be the mental state of the therapist when doing massage.

Indeed, the therapist would do well to have a constructive, healing attitude throughout the massage itself. As attitudes are translated into vibrations at a subtle level, the therapist influences the quality of his or her massage work with his or her thoughts. They must, therefore, have a healing mental attitude, not only when facilitating suggestive magnetic therapy, but also doing massage prior to magnetic healing.

Osteopaths

Of course, anyone could do suggestive magnetic therapy. But not everyone is qualified to diagnose and give specific physical suggestions to a body for its recovery. Osteopaths, because of their training and hands on practice of manipulation, are medically qualified, and their practice lends itself easily to magnetic healing. Thus, they may be in a most favorable situation to incorporate this healing into their treatments.

Both magnetic healing and spinal manipulations are done along the cerebrospinal system. The doctor could easily do magnetic healing and suggestion after spinal adjustments.

As the subject's or patient's confidence in the healer is important, doctors should rate highly in this respect. With such confidence, the healing facilitator's suggestions given to her patient during magnetic healing should be most effective because, when the conscious objective mind of the patient trusts (believes) the healer's suggestions, then the subconscious mind will accept them as true.

The doctor, with the ability to diagnose and prescribe, is able to formulate specific suggestions for a body's proper functioning and recovery. Suggestions used in suggestive magnetic therapy are to influence physical healing via the mind, while magnetic healing is used to influence the body mainly through the nervous system. It is the electromagnetic energy through the hands of the healer that directly affects the patient. Osteopaths, because of their hands-on practice, no doubt generate and radiate this energy to a high degree.

That this electromagnetic energy is a requirement and sustainer of life is not only a medical fact, but also acknowledged by physicists as well. Dr. M.Y. Han, in his book, *The Secret Life of Quanta,* states, *"Electric charges, whatever they are, and however they originated, are more than just fundamental. There is something almost sacred about them...Not only is electromagnetic radiation the life giver itself, it is nature's gift to us for microwave ovens, diagnostic x-rays, and telecommunications."*

The doctor, as well as the layperson, can enhance their magnetic healing treatments by acknowledging the role of electricity in life. That is, by thinking about electromagnetic energy radiating from their hands into the nerves and body of the patient as they perform these electrical treatments. Cayce emphasized the importance of electricity for healing in reading number 3266-1:

... Have the electrical treatments that may be applied to the body through the hands of the manipulator... These should be given by one making the adjustments osteopathically for the body.

... In giving the electrical treatment, let this be more along the spine and then the centers in the frontal portions of the body—as the patches of the lymph circulation, so that the glands of the abdomen and bowels and bladder are electrified through the centers themselves.

... If we do not electrify the body we are going to have much more disintegration.

Chiropractors

Chiropractors were mentioned many times in the Edgar Cayce readings. Because their practice mainly involves spinal adjustments, they, like osteopaths, would be likely facilitators for magnetic healing. It should be a simple matter to do such healing at the end of regular chiropractic treatments. This would require additional time of only ten minutes or so.

This Cayce reading encourages one chiropractor to include magnetic healing, adding that it would be materially profitable for her to do so.

(Q) What can I do in my present healing work [chiropractor] *to produce greater efficiency, both from my patient standpoint and from my own?*

(A) the natural tendencies and inclinations in the healing are such that, if the entity will use more and more of the magnetic forces of self, closer and closer may the entity come to be of a help to those who seek aid.

More and more use of those vibratory forces—as is understood—also brings material gain. For, again, it is not alone from the earth storehouses, but from the universal forces that strength of material natures may materialize in this experience for the entity. (1397-1)

Other Health Care Professionals

Physical therapists and nurses among others who do hands-on medical care should also make good suggestive magnetic therapists. Indeed, any healthcare professional who works directly with patients in a hands-on capacity could likely be magnetic healing facilitators.

To employ this healing in their work would require, of course, the approval of their superiors or employers. They would also require the diagnosis of a doctor if they are to effectively treat specific physical conditions.

More and more medical professionals are recognizing the effectiveness of spiritual involvement in physical wellness. Suggestive magnetic therapy is another spiritual healing method available to both the layperson and healthcare professional. It is an art that has been lost in time and medical advancements, but with renewed interest in the interaction of mind, body, and spirit, magnetic healing may once again play an important role in healing.

About Edgar Cayce

Edgar Cayce (1877-1945) has been called the "sleeping prophet," "the father of holistic medicine," and the most documented psychic of the 20th century. Cayce was born on a farm in Hopkinsville, Kentucky in 1877. His psychic abilities began to appear early in his childhood. As an adult, Cayce would put himself into a state of deep meditation, connecting with the Universal Consciousness, and from this state came his "readings." From holistic health and the treatment of illness to dream interpretation and reincarnation, Cayce's readings and insights offer practical help and advice to individuals from all walks of life, even today.

Discover the Edgar Cayce Material

The Association for Research and Enlightenment, Inc. (A.R.E.) was founded in 1931 by Edgar Cayce. Its international headquarters is in Virginia Beach, Virginia, where thousands of visitors come year-round. Many more are helped and inspired by A.R.E.'s local activities in their own hometowns, or by contact via email or regular mail with A.R.E. headquarters.

People all around the world have discovered meaningful and life-transforming insights in the A.R.E. programs and materials. These focus on such areas as personal spirituality, holistic health, dreams, family life, finding your best vocation, reincarnation, E.S.P., meditation, and soul growth in small group settings. You can call A.R.E. at its toll-free number: **1-800-333-4499**

or email: **http://www.edgarcayce.org**

You may also write or visit
A.R.E.
215 67th Street
Virginia Beach, VA 23451-2061

188

Sidney Weltmer and
The Weltmer Institute

——Δ——

Sidney Abrams Weltmer was born on July 7, 1858. Because of the lack of schools and teachers after the Civil War, he was basically home-schooled by this parents, both of whom were college educated.

By 1880 Weltmer was teaching and preaching in Tipton, Missouri. After his father died, he and his wife, Mary, moved to Atkinsville where he was instrumental in organizing school libraries in the county. He served as librarian until 1897 in the city of Selalia. Weltmer also taught mathematics and English at the local business college until 1895.

In 1895 Weltmer treated his first case. During the next two years he continued his studies and healing research while treating more than eight hundred people, most of whom could offer him no compensation. Favorable response to his efforts led him to move to Nevada, Missouri in 1897 where he established the Weltmer Institute that same year.

Following Weltmer's initiative, many "healers" and schools of healing soon made the town their base. Few, if any, had the sincerity, knowledge, and charisma of Sidney Weltmer for, by 1903, less than half a dozen remained in business.

The success of the Weltmer Institute was phenomenal. Not only were patients treated and Weltmer's healing methods taught in a four-year cource there, but the institute also offered distant healing and home-study correspondence courses.

The volume of mail directed to the Institute was so great that the town's post office was upgraded and enlarged. An increasing number of people came for treatments, requiring additional trains to meet the patients' transportation needs.

As with many innovative and pioneering practices, success brought envy, skepticism, and criticism. In 1899 Weltmer filed a slander suit against a minister. The case was won by Weltmer in the lower courts but was appealed by the defendant. Finally, the U.S. Supreme Court decided the case in Weltmer's favor, allowing graduates of the Weltmer Institutue's residence course to practice in any state. Still, the Court did require that a physician be on staff at the Institute to diagnose ailments, a requirement which Weltmer readily accepted. In fact, Ernest, Sidney Weltmer's oldest son became a medical doctor.

Visitors and patients came to the Institute from throughout the United States as well as from abroad. Yet, Sidney Weltmer never amassed a fortune. He was said to be civic-minded, contributed generously to charity drives, and was actively involved with the Elks, Masons, and other such organizations. The Institute continued to thrive for over thirty years, treating hundreds of thousands of patients at its Missouri headquarters, and more via "absentee treatments."

However, with the stock market crash and then the death of Sidney Weltmer on December 5, 1930 at age seventy-two, activities at the Weltmer Institute declined. Some of its staff attempted to carry on the work, but without the dynamic leadership of its founder, the Institute closed in the early 1930s.

Weltmer's widow wrote this farewell to her late husband in the December/January 1932 edition of *Weltmer's Magazine:*

This life which seems so important to most of us, which he, more than most men, realized was only an incident in eternal existence, is completed. The books are balanced and the account closed. As he did not begin with birth, and his eternal nature was not changed by the events of life, so he does not end with death.

Δ

For Further Study

Body Electric, The: Electromagnetism and the Foundation of Life, by Robert O. Becker, M.D., and Gary Selden, William Morrow and Company, 1985

Law of Psychic Phenomena, The, by Thomas Jay Hudson, Hudson-Cohan Publishing Co., 1925

Magnetic Healing (1901), *The Mystery Revealed* (1901), and *The Healing Hand* (1922), by Sidney A. Weltmer.

Medium, the Mystic, and the Physicist, The, by Lawrence LeShan, The Viking Press, 1974

Power of Your Subconscious Mind, The, by Joseph Murphy, D.R.S., D.D., Ph.D., LL.D, Prentice-Hall, Inc., 1963.

Vibrational Medicine, by Richard Gerber, M.D., Bear & Company, 1988

Your Mind: Unlocking Your Hidden Powers, by Henry Reed, Ph.D., A.R.E. Press, 1966

—